ADD WORLD
and the
ADDERALL
EXPLOSION

ADD WORLD
and the
ADDERALL
EXPLOSION

C Thomas Gualtieri MD

The Kenmore Press
Chapel Hill
2024
ISBN: 9798870242484

DEDICATION

For the pediatricians and primary care docs who aren't quite sure about ADD and stimulants but are trying to do the right thing.

CONTENTS

INTRODUCTION

What you have read and what you think you know about ADD and psychostimulant drugs is half-true. This book is about the other half.

My aim is to clear some of the confusion that exists about ADD and stimulant drugs like Ritalin and Adderall. A large, profitable industry has grown up around ADD, based on the dubious proposition that 10% of us have it. In the USA, about 4 million children and 11 million adults are prescribed stimulant drugs for ADD. To skeptics, that is horrifying. The converted worry that only half of all ADDs are ever treated at all.

ADD is said to afflict about 5% of people world-wide, but surveys in the USA show that 10% of children and adults take amphetamines for ADD. In some surveys, the rate is as high as 15%. There are schools where 30% of the children take a stimulant drug. And ADD is not just for kids anymore. Since 2014, more prescriptions for amphetamine have been written for adults than children.[1]

Every few years, they do a new survey. Every new survey shows more children and many more adults diagnosed with ADD and treated with stimulants.

The prevailing view is that ADD is a lifelong disorder, a genetic condition that runs in families. The cause is aberrant circuitry in the brain. The official view is that ADD is a 'neurodevelopmental disorder'.[2] There are strict criteria for the diagnosis. The problem is, the criteria are honored more in the breach than keeping. Most stimulant prescriptions are written for people who complain of mild problems with attention or mental fatigue.

We have to get a grip on this. We need to know what ADD really is and what it isn't. We know that stimulants are good for ADD patients but most stimulant prescriptions are written for people who aren't ADD.

Real ADD is a neurodevelopmental disorder that affects 1 or 2% of children and half as many adults. Most children diagnosed with ADD don't have the real thing. They are simply experiencing a transient developmental lag or they have an exuberant personality or an active, independent mind.

Real ADD is comparatively uncommon but ADD symptoms are ubiquitous. ADD symptoms occur in patients with anxiety or OC. They occur in adults with chronic fatigue or chronic pain, chemo-brain, long Covid and many chronic diseases. ADD symptoms may be signs of menopause or normal ageing. Difficulty concentrating is caused by overwork, sleep deprivation, deconditioning and stress. Nevertheless, such patients are told they have ADD. *Adult-onset ADD*, to be precise.

Is it really a danger to the public health if only half of all ADDs are ever treated? Untreated ADDs, they say, lose their jobs, get into car accidents and wind up in jail. Skeptics say that stimulants are dangerous drugs, that people get addicted and terrible things happen to them. There's a germ of truth on both sides, but extreme views are usually inaccurate and mostly irrelevant to those 15 million Americans who are prescribed amphetamines. They have many different kinds of problems. Calling them all ADDs deprives the diagnosis of all meaning. Providers and patients alike remain blind to that is really going on.

I started my career as a child psychiatrist treating ADD kids. Later, as a neuropsychiatrist, I've studied ADD in children and adults. I've written about ADD symptoms in patients with a number of different conditions, like brain injury and early dementia. Having observed the vigorous growth of ADD World over the past 50 years, I remain neither an advocate nor a skeptic. I think we all need to know what ADD is and what it isn't. We also need to understand what amphetamines do, for better or worse.

For example: stimulant drugs are *so safe we give them to children*. The dangers of low-dose stimulants in children and adolescents are often overstated. ADD children have been treated with amphetamines since the 1950s and we have yet to discover a long-term side-effect. However, the widespread use of stimulants by adults may not be so safe at all. I'm not going to reiterate all the problems that meth addicts and coke-heads have, but I will tell you that stimulants drugs are, to adults, cardiovascular risk factors. Are they as bad as high blood pressure, diabetes or smoking cigarettes? Maybe not, but we don't know.

I want to inject some common sense into ADD World. Mild problems with attention and mental fatigue are universal. Sometimes they cause difficulties that are more than mild. Problems with inattention, distractibility and self-regulation are not unique to ADD – they are prevalent among normal, healthy people. Problems with concentration and fatigue are so common that caffeine and nicotine, both mental stimulants, are the most widely consumed drugs in the world. When we give our NeuroPsych Questionnaire to normal, healthy people, they invariably describe mild problems with fatigue, anxiety, attention and memory.[*]

Amphetamine and methylphenidate happen to be more reliable and efficient mental stimulants than caffeine or nicotine. The two drugs improve attention and memory, increase energy and confer a state of well-being, all at the same time. When they are available, people like to take them. A lot of people. Does it surprise you?

I am going to tell you about the patients we see. We shall

---

[*] See for yourself; the NPQ is at www.atonc.com.

start with ADD as it was first described in 1947. It was originally a brain damage syndrome. Then we'll look at different kinds of children who are diagnosed with ADD and treated with stimulant drugs.

Adults who think they have ADD are a diverse group, too, even more so than kids. So, we shall meet adults with medical conditions like brain-fog and chemo-brain, who really need a stimulant. Then we shall meet healthy, normal people who take stimulants for their energizing, alerting effects, or for cognitive enhancement. Many of them do well enough but some don't.

This small book is about difficulties confronting clinicians who tend to those 15 million Americans and want to do the right thing.

A NOTE ABOUT TERMS

Why do I write **ADD** all the time when **ADHD** is the correct acronym? ADHD stands for Attention Deficit/Hyperactivity Disorder, but the older label was Attention Deficit Disorder, or ADD. I stick with ADD, and for good reason. It is euphonious; ADHD sounds like sneezing.[3]

The stimulant (or psychostimulant) drugs are Adderall, Dexedrine, Desoxyn and Ritalin. **Adderall** is a mixture of 'amphetamine salts' and is made up of d- and l-amphetamine. The d- and l- refer to different isomers, or variants, of the amphetamine molecule. A molecule is 'right-handed' (d) or 'left-handed' (l) depending on how it bends in three-dimensional space. The d-amphetamine isomer is more potent than the l-isomer, but the mix of d- and l-isomers in Adderall seems to have a more balanced effect. Commercial variants of Adderall are Mydayis and amphetamine salts.

The first amphetamine to be used clinically was **Benzedrine**, which was also a d- and l- mixture, but in a different proportion than Adderall. It is no longer available, but modern copies are Dyanavel, Evekeo, Adzenys, and amphetamine sulfate.

Dexedrine is pure d-amphetamine. Dexedrine is more potent than the d- and l- mixtures, especially on the neurotransmitter dopamine, while the latter have equal effects on dopamine and norepinephrine. Versions: Dexedrine, Vyvanse, Procentra, Xelstrym.

Desoxyn is methamphetamine (yes, meth) but it is rarely used for ADD. It is usually prescribed, if at all, for narcolepsy. It has a longer duration of action than Dexedrine or Adderall and is more toxic.

Ritalin is methylphenidate, not an amphetamine but structurally and functionally quite similar. It is not as potent as any of the amphetamines and has fewer side effects, especially in young children. It is less likely to be abused. Clinical variants of methylphenidate are Concerta, Focalin, Metadate, Quillivant, Quillichew, Adhansia, Aptensio, Cotempla, Daytrana, Jornay, and Methylin.

Sometimes I use **amphetamines** to refer to all the stimulants, including Ritalin. For example, 'Amphetamines have been around for a long time: Benzedrine (1932), Dexdedrine (1937), methamphetamine (1938), Ritalin (1954) and Adderall (1994).' I should have said 'Stimulant drugs have been around…' but one gets tired of writing 'stimulant' all the time.

The little numbers you see in the text, like [1], [2], [3], [4], etc. refer to notes at the end of the book. The numbers are sequential, starting with [1] and we're already up to [4].

PART ONE

ADD IN CHILDREN

If you want to understand ADD and the explosion of amphetamine prescription, you have to know how it all started. Before we get to ADD in adults, I shall explain what ADD is in children.

My explanations are based on the different patients we see at our clinics. We shall meet Martin and Felix who were ADD, for sure, and who had a lifetime of problems. But they represent only a small minority of children diagnosed with ADD. Then there is Henry, whose ADD was a reflection of his exuberant personality. High energy and impatience made trouble for him in school but they will be assets when he grows up. Carrie and Tim had transient ADD symptoms when they were confronted with developmental challenges they weren't ready for. There are ten such children for every 5 Henrys and every one Martin. If they require stimulant treatment, it only for a short time, no more than 2 or 3 years.

Cam had an active mind and high energy but he was creative and imaginative. Schoolwork wasn't as interesting to him as what was going on inside his head.

When we get to adults with ADD, or self-proclaimed ADD, some will resemble the children we've met, but they are a more diverse group. Growing up makes it easier for us to make problems for ourselves.

1. ADD USED TO BE MBD

Not too long ago, when I began my career as a child psychiatrist, this is what ADD was like:

> Martin was 8 years old when I met him. He couldn't sit still. He bounced around the examining room and his parents had to restrain him on the couch. He didn't do well in school. He wouldn't stay in his seat so the teacher made him sit right next to her desk so she could control him. If she took her eyes off him, he would be up again, making mischief. His attention span was seconds-long.
>
> Matin's IQ was on the low side of average and he had trouble learning to read. He had an IEP – an individualized education plan – for ADD and dyslexia. He was a good-natured child but impulsive, and he constantly got into things. He broke his arm when he jumped off the balcony; it wasn't his only misadventure. He didn't do well with other kids because he was too wild. He couldn't play sports because of his undisciplined nature but he was also clumsy and poorly coordinated. Nevertheless, he couldn't resist climbing anything that could possibly be climbed and some things you never thought could be. He only fell a few times. He might have had a few concussions but you wouldn't know it if he did because he'd shake them off. Then he was up and running again...

We didn't call it ADD then, or ADHD. It was minimal brain dysfunction, or MBD.

Martin's parents were normal, working-class people. His mother stayed home and his father was a retired Marine. They were kind and attentive parents and he was their only son. They tried never to be rough with him, but it wasn't always possible. They were frustrated and perplexed.

The pregnancy was normal but the delivery was difficult and he had to be resuscitated at birth. He grew quickly but his development was a bit slow. As soon as he could walk, he ran.

In spite of frequent accidents, Martin was a healthy child. He had difficulty on almost all the tests we gave him because he wouldn't pay attention. He also had difficulty reading. He would get letters mixed up: b for d, i for j, m for n. He wrote letters backwards, too. He didn't like going to bed. He thrived on a few hours of sleep.

The examination was not quite normal and it took a while because he wouldn't sit still on the examining table and kept grabbing the stethoscope and the reflex hammer. He was clearly hyperactive, impulsive and inattentive. He had a number of neurological soft signs, minor signs of neurological immaturity, and several minor physical anomalies.[4]

We treated Martin with Ritalin and later with Dexedrine. He responded, not especially well, but he wasn't quite so hyperactive or distractible. He still had difficulties at school and dropped out when he was 16.

I kept up with Martin because his father decided that he, too, had ADD. When he came for periodic visits, he told me about his son. Martin never bothered to take medications again. He tried to join the Marines but was rejected. He had one job after another, sometimes two at a time. He married a woman who was ten years older, with two children. She said that Martin was her third child.

I met him, by chance, at an equipment store where he worked. He was as happy and energetic as ever and ran to the back to get me what I was looking for. He came back in a jiffy, almost running. He brought me the wrong thing.

That is what ADD used to be like, when it was MBD. They were called hyperactive children and it wasn't hard to make the diagnosis. MBD kids are hyper everywhere, including the examining room, and Martin is a good example. In addition to all the hallmarks of ADD, he was poorly coordinated and had a learning disability and an abnormal neurological exam.

MBD was originally Minimal Brain Damage. The concept evolved during the 1940s from studies of children who had suffered brain injuries, brain infections or obstetrical accidents. Some were survivors of the encephalitis pandemic in 1917-28.* Many of the children who survived the virus were hyperactive, distractible, irritable, unruly, and unmanageable in school. The children were said to have 'Mild Brain Damage', MBD. The few child psychiatrists and pediatric neurologists who tended to such children realized that they resembled the veterans of World War I who had suffered traumatic brain injuries. The soldiers were studied by a German neuropsychiatrist, Kurt Goldstein. Brain damage, Goldstein said, led to 'a general loss of inhibitory control'. They had problems with self-regulation or self-control, especially notable when the injury was to the frontal lobes of the brain, the *prefrontal cortex* (PFC) in particular. The injured veterans were said to have the *Frontal Lobe Syndrome*. Today, we call it *Executive Dysfunction* and the *Central Executive* resides in the prefrontal cortex.

(If you want to know where your frontal lobes are, here's how. Lay the heel of your hand on your forehead, right over your eyebrows, and spread your fingers as you lay your hand on the scalp. If you have an average head and an average-sized hand, the frontal lobes are beneath it, on the inside of your head, of course. Your fingers are above the motor and premotor cortices, which govern movement. Your palm overlies the prefrontal cortex, the seat of self-regulation, behavior control, judgment, motivation and deep thought; they are called the

---

* Oliver Sacks' Book, Awakenings, is about survivors of that epidemic.

executive functions. The development of the frontal lobes is a long and arduous process; the myelination of frontal neurons, for example, is not completed in humans until the fifth decade of life. It is ironic that frontal lobe maturation is not complete until after core rot has set in below.[5])

Goldstein's observations held sway during the 1940s and 50s. Then, in the 1960s, physicians observed that problems with hyperactivity, emotional dysregulation and inattention also occurred in children who had not suffered overt brain injury. The term Mild or Minimal Brain Damage was replaced by Minimal Brain *Dysfunction.* The new term retained the euphonious acronym, MBD, and was less harsh. MBD kids were hyperactive and distractible, and the diagnosis required an examination to reveal signs or incoordination or neurological immaturity (soft signs) and testing to show learning disabilities or delays in language development.

During the 1960s, only a few physicians knew about MBD. The diagnosis was usually made by a pediatric neurologist or a developmental pediatrician. (Linda Blair's mother took her to a neurologist at Georgetown, and he prescribed Ritalin.[†]) In fact, it was Ritalin and Dexedrine that attracted attention to MBD, and those drugs weren't used very much until the 60s. The therapeutic effects were remarkable. Kids with MBD learned better and had fewer behavior problems. The drugs were remarkably safe.

In 1968, the American Psychiatric Association decided that MBD was a mental disorder. They changed the name to the 'Hyperkinetic Reaction of Childhood'. In 1980, they changed it again, to Attention Deficit Disorder (ADD) and again in 1987, to Attention Deficit/Hyperactivity Disorder'. The euphonious acronym was changed as well, from MBD to ADD and then ADHD.

The terms minimal brain damage or dysfunction were

[†] The Exorcist, remember?

abandoned because they were thought to be impossibly vague. It was impossible to demonstrate exactly what kind of 'brain dysfunction' might account for the problems of hyperactive kids. Yet MBD children are different. They are only a small minority of the children who are currently diagnosed with ADD. They have a much higher rate of learning disabilities. Ironically, they respond less well to psychostimulants and even with the best treatments their problems persist. Their futures, too, are clouded. They are much more likely to have difficulties in adult life: unsuccessful marriages, chronic unemployment and problems with the law.

In 1968, ADD was unmoored from its neurological underpinnings and was now a mental disorder – a *neurodevelopmental disorder*, to be precise. The diagnosis was based on the presence of "overactivity, restlessness, distractibility, and short attention span."[‡] It wasn't necessary for a physician to observe signs of the condition or even test for them. The diagnosis could be made on the basis of what parents and teachers *said* about the child. There was no need for a physical or neurological exam or cognitive testing. In the 1970s, the numbers of children diagnosed with 'hyperkinesis' began to climb and they haven't stopped.

Today, the diagnosis of ADD is no longer restricted, as it once was, to children with neurological deficits, minor physical anomalies, uncontrollable behavior problems and school failure. The diagnosis has been broadened to include many different types of children and even more adults. Their sole complaint is difficulty concentrating on school or work.[§]

[‡] From the DSM-II, in 1968: "308.0. Hyperkinetic reaction of childhood (or adolescence). This disorder is characterized by overactivity, restlessness, distractibility, and short attention span, especially in young children; the behavior usually diminishes in adolescence. If this behavior is caused by organic brain damage, it should be diagnosed under the appropriate non-psychotic organic brain syndrome."

The problem with ADD is not its name or the theories behind it. It is that the symptoms of ADD are so prevalent in children and adults. More than 50% of children are said to have short attention spans, according to their teachers, and more than 50% of boys are said to be overactive by their mothers.[6]

The symptoms of ADD are also non-specific. They occur in normal healthy children, in kids with ADD, and in kids with all sorts of other problems. If the diagnosis of ADD is based simply on what a parent, teacher or patient *says*, then a lot of people are going to be ADD. That is exactly what happened.

---

§ By that standard, we are *all* ADD.

2. AMPHETAMINES FOR CHILDREN?

The number of children taking a stimulant drug for the Hyperkinetic Syndrome increased threefold during the 1970s. Slowly but surely, physicians grew comfortable with the idea of prescribing stimulants to children. This is an example of ADD as we knew it then:

> Felix was seven when his mother complained to her pediatrician. The child was overactive, restless and distractible. He had always been active, even as a baby, and he was a restless sleeper. He woke up early and was ready to go, usually around 6 am. He was a good kid but he got in trouble at school for bothering the other children. He couldn't sit still. His teacher asked his mother if he might be ADD. So, Rachel asked her pediatrician.

> She (the pediatrician) knew that Felix was a healthy kid. He was smart enough; he had always passed his developmental screenings. She gave Rachel a rating scale to fill out and one for his teacher to do. She also suggested that Rachel and her husband attend parenting classes with a psychologist who was attached to the office.

> The rating scales came back and his scores indicated ADD. He got a prescription for Ritalin. Felix' insurance wouldn't cover the psychologist, but his parents didn't really need the behavior management classes. Rachel and Lorne both came from big families and Felix was their third child. They knew how to manage behavior. They just couldn't manage Felix.

What drove the extraordinary increase in ADD diagnosis was the availability of a safe, effective and inexpensive treatment. The pediatrician told Rachel that stimulants are safe; millions of children have been treated with amphetamine and methylphenidate for more than 70 years and we have yet to discover a negative long-term side effect.[7] Stimulants do have a number of nasty short-term side effects: dysphoria, loss of appetite and weight loss, GI distress, headache, motor and phonic tics.[8] Some children are so suppressed when they take a stimulant they are like zombies. The good thing about stimulant side effects, though, is that they are readily apparent; a conscientious parent will stop the drug right away.

Stimulants are effective, too; you can see how effective they are an hour after the child gets a test dose.[9] Within an hour, patients are visibly more attentive and perform better on cognitive tests. There are arguments about exactly how effective stimulants are over the long-term, and we shall visit that topic later. However, the short-term effects of psychostimulant drugs are undeniable: they improve attention and reduce hyperactivity and impulsiveness in children. In adults they have immediate effects on alertness and energy.

Nevertheless, one has to acknowledge that administering psychoactive drugs to children is an extraordinary thing to do. The child's brain is a moving target. Between birth and puberty, it is developing at an astonishing rate; cortical connections are being made and neural networks are being set down. How do stimulant drugs affect all that, or any of the other drugs we feed to children? Prescribing a medication that may influence these delicate processes is a special undertaking.

We routinely administer potent medications to children for a 'disorder' characterized by high energy, impetuosity and a disinclination towards dull, boring work. Do we really know what we are doing? Has anyone read Tom Sawyer?

Amphetamines for *children*? Where did that idea come from?

By accident, actually.   In 1928, Benzedrine was the first American stimulant, a mixture of d- and l-amphetamine, and the manufacturer was determined to find a use for it.   The company, Smith, Kline and French, thought it might be good for nasal congestion.   Then, in 1935, they made it available to physicians to explore its stimulating effects on brain function. Before long, physicians were giving Benzedrine to patients with fatigue or mild depression.   University students began using it as a cognitive enhancer.

Charles Bradley was one of those physicians. He had trained in pediatrics and neurology at Columbia.   Once finished, he was recruited to direct a psychiatric treatment center for children in Rhode Island; it had been founded by his great-uncle who named it the Bradley Home after his disabled daughter.   When Dr Bradley received his first supply of Benzedrine, he used it to treat headache. Bradley was in the habit of doing spinal taps on the children in the Home; they were a mix of kids with behavior problems and mental illness, but many had subtle neurological abnormalities (i.e., MBD), so an EEG and lumbar puncture seemed reasonable things to do. After the LP, most kids had headache, so Bradley gave them Benzedrine.   It didn't help the headache, but the kids did better at the hospital school; they called it their 'math pills'. So informed by the teachers, Bradley followed up and reported that about half the children treated with Benzedrine improved their school performance and also their impulsive behavior.

Bradley's patients were a diverse group of children with behavior disorders, emotional problems, autism and psychosis. Even allowing for the diagnostic imprecision of the day, Bradley's observations indicated that the effects of amphetamine were not limited to any single category of patient. The psychotic children responded almost as well as the kids with emotional or behavior problems.

Stimulant treatment was one of those occasional events in medicine – like quinine, colchicine, reserpine and digitalis – where a successful treatment is discovered long before physicians had any idea what it is they are treating. Bradley had stumbled across a relatively non-specific treatment that happened to improve attention and impulse control in children with a variety of different problems. He didn't associate amphetamine treatment with any particular diagnosis; MBD wasn't even recognized until ten years later.

Bradley's papers, published in 1937 and 1939, had virtually no impact. It wasn't until the 1950s that Bradley's work was acknowledged. When it was, the circle closed and the therapeutic benefits of amphetamine were linked to MBD.

Diagnosis and treatment thus found each other. The relatively non-specific nature of the stimulant response that Bradley had observed was supplanted by specific prescription for MBD. Bradley's description of beneficial effects with amphetamine was affirmed in 1967 when the first controlled study of d-amphetamine (Dexedrine) was published, in children with the Hyperkinetic syndrome.[10]

In the 1970s, neuroscientists took a special interest in childhood hyperactivity because of what they thought was a 'paradoxical response'. Children like Martin and Felix calmed down when they took amphetamine while adults who took the drug speeded up. It was a neuropharmacological conundrum that could be replicated in laboratory animals. Scientists could make young rats hyperactive, usually by damaging their nervous systems with a neurotoxin like lead or carbon monoxide, and the rats would quiet down after they were given a small dose of amphetamine. When the rats grew up, amphetamine made them run around like crazy. At the time, this was a compelling focus of argument and discussion. Some clinicians, in a triumph of circular reasoning, proposed that a positive behavioral response to stimulants affirmed the diagnosis of Hyperkinetic Syndrome.

That's when I got involved. I was finishing my fellowship in child psychiatry and had the privilege of joining a research project that aimed to address difficult problems. There were plenty of problems to solve: whether stimulant treatment stunted a child's growth, whether it was useful to measure blood levels of Ritalin, and what happened to hyperactive children when they were given antipsychotic drugs, which happened all-too-frequently in those days.[11] The paradoxical response to stimulants, however, was resolved by other researchers, who showed that normal children responded to amphetamine; and then that normal adults responded to methylphenidate just as hyperactive children did.[12] They slowed down and paid attention. The 'paradoxical response' had put ADD on the scientific map. Yet it was a fallacy. Then, too, was the idea that response to amphetamine was specific to ADD.

We should have known better.

The cognitive effects of amphetamine were common knowledge by the nineteen-forties, when it widely used by the military. Mostly it was used to counter fatigue in soldiers and pilots. The US Navy gave it to men who operated SONAR devices on ships in the battle of the North Atlantic. With a small dose of Benzedrine, sailors were able to attend to the screen for longer periods of time, they were less distractible, less vulnerable to the fatigue induced by a boring task, and they made fewer omission errors. That is, they didn't miss so many submarines. Benzedrine saved countless thousands of lives because psychostimulants improve almost everyone's ability to sustain attention to dull, boring tasks. The response of hyperactive kids wasn't paradoxical at all. We should have known.[13]

3. ADD IS A PERSONALITY TRAIT

ADD is a neurodevelopmental disorder, defined as such by the American Psychiatric Association. The definition is supported by 80 years of research and thousands of research papers in medical journals. Martin fit the bill and Felix did, too.

In fact, ADD is not just a neurodevelopmental disorder, and sometimes it's not a disorder at all. It's different things. What we call ADD is different in different people. In a lot of kids, it's a 'disorder' only because we look at more-or-less-normal human weaknesses as disorders.

> Henry was 10 years old, healthy, happy and smart enough. He had always been an active little boy and he loved sports. He liked school because his friends were there but his teachers complained he would talk out in class and was rambunctious. He hated to do homework and if he finished an assignment, he would lose it or forget to turn it in. He made careless mistakes, his attention span was short and he never seemed to listen.
>
> *He's just like his father*, said his mother. *His mother said he was just like that in school.* She and Henry senior were happily married, and they had a second child, a little girl who must have been just like her mother because she was well-behaved and loved school. Maryanne, Henry's mother, had to leave her job and take over the books for the contracting business, which was successful but about to go bust because Henry senior couldn't keep up with the paperwork.
>
> Henry was, indeed, a healthy, happy kid, and his neurological exam was normal. His gross motor

skills were exceptional – he could even skip backwards. His testing showed normal intelligence and he did well on every test except two tests of attention. We gave him a test dose of Ritalin and the family went to lunch.

When they came back an hour later, Henry was quiet but not subdued. His heart rate and blood pressure hadn't changed. He took the tests again and aced them. We gave him a prescription for long-acting Ritalin. A month later, Maryanne reported that his schoolwork had improved 100%, and there were no more complaints about talking out in class or bothering other children. He took Ritalin for the rest of the term but he didn't take it again until High School.

Henry took Ritalin for a while, and then he caught on to what he had to do to get by. He didn't need it until 12th grade. In High School he was into sports, girls and his friends, and working for his father on his days off. He played football and baseball. He bought his first car by himself when he was 16. He needed Ritalin one more time, when he was a senior and had to pass math to graduate. Then he went to community college, where he did well without Ritalin because he was studying construction. Then he joined his father's business. He will take it over someday. Hopefully he will marry someone who can keep the books.

Henry was diagnosed with ADD a couple of times and treated with Ritalin twice. It did the job, both times. So, he was ADD. But was he? Did he really have a neurodevelopmental disorder or brain dysfunction? I don't think so. He had a few weaknesses that were part of his personality. In Henry, and his father, what we call ADD is just the way they are.

Henry and his father had symptoms of ADD, but they had

perfectly healthy brains. Didn't they have a math disability? Maybe, but I think it was just disinterest in academic math. They could calculate the pitch of a roof and how many board-feet it would take to build a deck. They were both strong and well-coordinated. They could read people really well and they both had a lot of friends. They would both get mad, usually for a good reason, but they got over it quickly. Maryanne would agree that they both were impulsive (impetuous), hyperactive (high energy) and inattentive (easily bored) but she didn't think they had a neurodevelopmental disorder or brain dysfunction. She knew she had a strong, loyal and hard-working husband and a strong, devoted and hard-working son. They were resilient, cheerful and always busy. They both could make her laugh.

Henry senior was a successful builder. He employed a lot of people and could concentrate on several projects at the same time. When construction took a downturn, which it does periodically, he tried to keep his crews busy and ate the loss. If he were a corporate executive, he would have laid them all off. But you can't say he had 'executive dysfunction'. He had values. He had motivation, initiative and persistence, he learned from his mistakes, responded appropriately to rewards and punishment and could defer gratification. Boy, could he delay gratification. It's why his wife quit her job at the hospital and took over billing for his company.

Henry senior had been like his son when he was in school. He had even been treated with Ritalin when he was a kid but he hated it.

If Henry and his father had brain dysfunction or a neurodevelopmental disorder, it's only because we label certain personality traits and cognitive styles as such. All of us have strengths and weaknesses but not every weakness deserves to be deemed pathological.

In a good many children who are thought to be ADD, their high energy and disinterest in schoolwork is a reflection of their personalities. The irony is that stimulants work as well, or better, when they are used to compensate normal human weaknesses. This, BTW, is why so many adults are said to be ADD.

Henry's ADD was an expression of his personality. It was the way he was.

Personality is who we are. It is an individual's unique style of thinking, feeling, acting and responding. It is composed of traits, behavioral, emotional and cognitive traits. A person is extraverted or introverted, calm or worrisome, agreeable or surly, etc. Some of us are active and energetic while others are passive and indolent. Some people are excitable, others phlegmatic. Some are bold, others shy, and so on. Cognitive traits are the way we think. Some of us are impulsive and act without thinking whilst others are reflective and cautious. Some are quick and others dull. Some of us have active minds that demand to be engaged. Other minds are content to wander idly and daydream.

These were some of Henry's traits, and his father's: they were impetuous, not cautious, but they were perfectionists when construction was involved. They were quick to react, not inhibited. They were high-spirited and loved to be engaged in something stimulating. For Henry, it was sports, girls and helping his Father on days out of school. For his Father, it was building sturdy houses, preferably several at the same time. Henry and his father had individual cognitive styles. They were intuitive, not reflective. They could hone in on matters that were important but were impatient with irrelevant details. They liked challenges. Henry's father loved to build something new and different.

We all know what personality is, but psychologists weren't content to leave it there. They wanted to make a science of it. They started a hundred years ago when two of them decided to study it in a systematic way. They took a bottom-up approach. This they took to be Webster's dictionary and so they counted every adjectives that describes a human characteristic. They found 17,953 such words, including *wowf, Byronic, pubigerous* and *cactiform*. In fact, it wasn't the psychologists who did the looking, but "three anonymous people" and I bet they were paid by the word and made some of them up.

Rather than concede that there were at least 17,953 human traits – and I think that's a bare minimum – the two psychologists started honing the list, combining words that meant the same thing and eliminating some, like wowf and cactiform, that I wish they had left in. They got the list of human traits down to 4504, and successive generations of psychologists honed the list further. Applying ever more clever statistical manipulations, they reduced the number of relevant adjectives to ten, which, in an uncharacteristic burst of colloquialism they call the Big Five.[14]

That doesn't mean that all of us have just ten characteristics, although I met some people who have fewer than that. But this isn't the time to talk about my immediate family. In fact, the Big Five are *dimensions* of personality with, for example, extraverted on one end of the spectrum and introverted on the other. Everyone is somewhere on the spectrum and usually a mix, extraverted sometimes and introverted at other times. The advantage of the Big Five is that it allows combinations and permutations of human characteristics that are virtually infinite, which brings us full circle back to those 17,953 adjectives. So much for personality science.

ADD just needs three adjectives to describe its tribe: distractible, hyperactive and impulsive. That leaves 17,950 more adjectives to determine whether a presumed ADD has a disorder or is pretty much normal.

Distractibility is a symptom. It is also a cognitive trait: impatience with topics that are not engaging. When their minds are not engaged, ADD kids are easily distracted. They don't necessarily have a short attention span; ADD kids can stay ensconced in a videogame for hours. Henry was impatient with differential equations. But he could work 12 hours straight framing a house.

Hyperactivity is a symptom. It is also the behavioral trait of high energy. ADD kids have a lot of energy and a bit of difficulty restraining themselves. They are, after all, children. As they grow up, high energy is a distinct advantage. When they get old, it keeps them active and healthy. Henry *pére & fils* were successful because they were high-energy.

Excitability is a symptom. It's like impulsivity, reacting sharply and suddenly to events. It is also a emotional trait, to feel strongly about things and express oneself accordingly. It's not a bad way to motivate a crew when they are lagging on a job.

Symptoms are from disorders, illnesses, diseases. Personality traits are the way people are. Traits are normally distributed in the population. That means that the frequency with which they occur is represented by a bell (normal) curve. For any particular trait, most of us cluster around the middle of the bell curve. ADD children are in the end (the 'tail') of the distribution in traits like high energy, quick to react and easily bored.

ADD, then is just math. It's where you are on the bell curve. Henry was to the left of the mean. Martin, in contrast, was far out in the tail of the curve. Felix was somewhere between.

In most cases, ADD is a constellation of personality traits. That fits three known facts. One is that ADD is a 'genetic condition'; personality traits and cognitive styles tend to run in families. The second is that ADD 'symptoms' often persist into adult life; personality traits are more-or-less stable. When I remember the third I'll let you know.[15]

4. THEY ARE CAVE-MEN, GONE ASTRAY

I am not an expert on personality by any means. I gave mine up years ago. But I have observed that ethnic, racial and religious differences are nothing compared to how diverse human personalities are. Every one of us, like it or not, has a unique personality. You are the one and only who perceives and reacts to things the way you do. Deal with it.

Nature knew what She was doing when She made us that way. It is likely that we humans evolved as quickly as we did, most of us anyway, because of our diverse behavioral characteristics. Natural selection likes diversity; it gives it something to work with. In fact, personality is the single biggest determinant of human mate selection. We experience personality, the way we and others are, and we react intuitively. We don't need adjectives to fall in love or know to avoid someone assiduously.

To belabor the point, compare the human being to one of his closest relatives, the chimpanzee. Since this book is meant to be read aloud to the whole family, I won't refer to chimpanzee mating habits. I shall choose a less savory example. Every chimp reacts to a clump of bananas in the same way. They eat as many as they can, burp and go to sleep. In contrast, humans are astonishingly diverse in their approach to the banana. Some like them green and others wait until they are brown. They might eat the squishy things or make them into delicious cakes, fritters, muffins, pies, pancakes or pudding, fried bananas and *bananas Foster*, for heaven's sake. Some people eat a banana from the flower tip (the distal end) and others from the neck. Some humans dislike bananas and there are people who make sure they eat one every morning. Someone I knew in college was afraid of bananas because, when she was a child, her grandfather told her that venomous snakes hid among the bunches. (He was very old and had a cruel sense of humor. His bad jokes outlived him.) Shy diabetics avoid bananas because of their high glycemic index and bold diabetics eat banana splits. Some people are indifferent to bananas and wonder if they are a fit subject for a scientific tome such as this. My friend Miles once said, *I can take them or leave them alone.* I, myself, have moderate views of the banana, but you may not be interested in my preferences just now. The point is that humans are so diverse, their differences are manifest even in regard to a small yellow fruit.

Human diversity serves us well. George Orwell once said something like this: *We sleep soundly in our beds because rough men stand ready in the night to visit violence on those who would do us harm.* Orwell was writing during the dark days of the Battle of Britain, when rough men cleared the skies and protected England from invasion. We 21st century aesthetes ought to remember the importance of rough men and women, and not only in wartime.

Some of us like to get our hands dirty and faces smudged with grease. There has to be somebody to sweep the street or empty septic tanks just as there has to be someone who likes to pontificate to disinterested undergraduates. Some of us spend our days adding up numbers. Some of us come home from the office at a reasonable hour, share a dinner of quinoa and salmon patties from Whole Foods and spend the evening watching PBS. Henry senior usually gets home around nine, eats a cold dinner, hands the day's bills to his wife and collapses in bed.

Diversity is more than a 21st century catchword. Nature has known about it for years.[16]

In that vein, there is a theory that ADD is a holdover from the days when human beings tramped across the savannah. They survived because some were good hunters and strong warriors. The theory proposes that qualities of such rough men are ADD symptoms: to scan the environment constantly, to be alert to every sight and sound, to hyperfocus in intense situations and to react quickly when they have to. Theoretically, ADDs are holdovers from the paleolithic. That doesn't explain why there are more ADDs around now than there were 50 years ago, of course, unless something has unleashed a generation of atavistic throwbacks.*

According to the theory, Martin, Felix, Henry and his Dad and even your sweet little daughter, who teachers say has trouble paying attention, are just cave-persons who were born in the wrong epoch. It is the 'mismatch theory' of ADD. Our ADDs, in all their millions, are poorly matched to the knowledge economy and would be better served if we let them form into small bands and released them into a game reserve.

I am not one to hold forth on the habits of prehistoric hunters and warriors. I've never even met a hunter-gatherer, and I doubt many of you have, either. That's why it's easy for theorizers to relate present-day problems to our prehistoric past. If that theorizer had spent time in the depths of the Amazon or the Kalahari Desert and was speaking with authority, I might take her theory seriously. Nevertheless, I would respond that ADD traits are equally adaptive for builders, elite athletes, Wall Street predators and arbitrageurs, travelling salesmen, trapeze artists, muleskinners and underwater welders, none of whom, I think, were around during the stone-age. Also, I wonder if ADDs make good hunters at all. As Dr Tiolo said, *I question whether I would want to go hunting in a terrain that includes lions, venomous reptiles, and other dangerous animals with someone who may be impulsive, disorganized, and accident-prone.*[17]

---

*Now that's not something you hear every day: *atavistic throwback*. It means the emergence of a primitive characteristic in a modern organism. I thought you might like a new phrase you can use, someday, to describe someone you don't like. It's not in the Urban Dictionary but it was among Gordon Allport's 17,953 adjectives.

The cave-man theory is a diversion, but it underscores the point that the symptoms of ADD are not necessarily symptoms at all but rather human personality traits. This accounts for Henry and his father and a good many ADD children and adults. Henry and his father had traits that are misinterpreted as ADD symptoms. Drs Ratey and Hallowell described those traits well: *high energy, creativity, intuitiveness, resourcefulness, tenacity, a love for hard work, a never-say-die approach, warm-heartedness, a trusting and forgiving attitude, sensitivity, the ability to take risks, flexibility, and a good sense of humor.* Those traits, BTW, do not typify our MBDs.

The wide range of human diversity includes those who are reflective and others who are quick to react. In fact, such 'symptoms' of ADD are ubiquitous in Nature. Sunfish, for example. There are bold sunfish and shy ones. Drop pieces of bread in a pond. The sunfish will gather around. Then one or two will swim forth and grab a piece of bread. They are the bold ones. Then a few more, and then the whole bunch. The shy ones are the last to venture forth and are left with only a few crumbs. The shy ones will die out, you'd think, but they don't. If the bread pieces were actually bait on a hook, it's the bold sunfish who would perish. The world community of sunfish thrives because it includes individuals with diverse traits. If someone were to bother, I bet the traits of boldness and shyness in sunfish could be plotted on a normal curve.

Then there is a passerine bird, *parus major,* the great tit. If you didn't know, great tits are a diverse bunch. For example, there are great tits who are bold, highly reactive, aggressive and quick to find good things to eat. On the other side, there are shy tits, who tend to be cautious and reflective. They keep to the undergrowth and scratch about, finding food in unlikely places. There is a balance between the two. Bold tits thrive when food is plentiful but are at a loss when food is scarce. They are also more vulnerable to predators. Shy tits, in contrast, do well during times of scarcity, knowing where to find a juicy seed secreted in the bush. They also escape the notice of owls and hawks.

There are other deviant qualities among the great tits but I've made my point and wont regale you with more stories from the *haunts of coot and hern*. In Nature, species succeed when they include individuals with diverse traits and personality differences among the animals can't compare to the diversity of our species. Humans, arguably the most successful species of all, are also the most diverse in terms of personality traits and cognitive styles. During the five million years of our evolution, it has given natural selection a lot to work with.

Evolution has landed us humans in an interesting place. There are bold, impetuous humans and shy, reflective ones. Some of us are wide-open and others cautious and closed-up. Some of us never worry and others are uptight. I don't think that natural selection is going to choose one type over the other anytime soon, but you never know. If we continue to hype up the first group with amphetamines, you don't know what's going to happen.

Martin and Henry teach us two things about the condition formerly known as ADD. In some people ADD is the consequence of brain injury or abnormal development. In others, it is constellation of personality traits and cognitive styles that are handicapping in some situations and advantageous in others.

With Martin we learned that the prefrontal cortex is large and complex, and very important, but it is also vulnerable to insults, that is, damage from many causes, great or small. With Henry, we learn that the front parts of brain are the seat of many of our personality traits and cognitive styles. The size and complexity of the human prefrontal cortex is the source of many if not most of the differences we humans share. It is large and complex region, with innumerable connections that form in accordance with one's genes, with experiences and also, just to keep matters interesting, at random. Everyone has a PFC that is different from everyone else's. In spite of the fact that your second ex-husband probably had the same bad habits your first did, we humans are all unique and everyone is different.

Bananas, OTOH, are pretty much all the same.

5. DYSMATURATION

The thing formerly known as ADD is something yet again. Now, meet Carrie, who has a completely different kind of ADD.

> She was 13 years old. She was bright, healthy and active. She had always done well in school, but her grades started to go down in 7th grade.   She had never been a behavior problem. She was a smart kid, but her grades went from all As to mostly Bs and a C in math. She told her parents she needed Ritalin. When we met her, she was polite and well-spoken.

> Carrie's examination was perfectly normal but the child and her parents cited problems with attention and memory. Neurocognitive testing showed mild problems with attention on two tests. We gave Carrie a test dose of Ritalin and she returned to clinic an hour later. She felt no different and her vital signs didn't change at all. But her attention tests improved to normal.

> We gave the child prescriptions for Concerta and Adderall to compare. She returned a month later; she preferred Concerta because Adderall affected her appetite.

> We treated her with Concerta and her grades improved. She took the med on school days and went off it on weekends and holidays. She did well. Two years later, she stopped the drug and continued to do well at school. She never had an adverse effect.

Carrie had problems with sustained attention and was performing below her ability in school. She responded to a stimulant and did well after she was treated. But was she really ADD? She was, if you stretch the diagnostic criteria a bit. The criteria are conservative. According to the DSM:

- ADD symptoms have to have been present before age 12. Carrie was 13, but her mother said, *She never liked to study but she never had to. Last year she had to apply himself for the first time.* Check.
- The symptoms have to occur in two or more settings. *She can't focus at school or homework.* Check.
- There must be "clear evidence" that the symptoms are disabling. Are Bs and Cs really disabling? Carrie's parents were worried that if she didn't get better grades this year she wouldn't qualify for the advanced program in High School. She would lose interest school, get into drugs, etc. Check, maybe.

When children like Carrie are diagnosed with ADD, it is because the diagnostic criteria are being applied loosely. Clinicians are known to stretch diagnostic boundaries. Judicious physicians may confer the diagnosis when diagnostic criteria aren't met, because even 'subclinical' disorders cause difficulty. Plus, insurance doesn't pay if the patient doesn't have a diagnosis.

For every Martin we meet in the clinic, there are at least five Henrys and more than ten Carries. The irony of stimulant treatment is that the drugs work well in milder cases, often better than they do in the Martins of the world.

Martin, Felix, Henry and Carrie (maybe) were all ADD. But they were different. ADD, it seems, includes children with different problems. Do they all fit in the same pigeonhole? It would be one that accommodated an awfully big pigeon.

ADD is an umbrella that covers many different kinds of people. The most common cause of ADD symptoms is what Carrie had: *dysmaturation*. That means that her development was behind normative expectations. But just the development of her regulatory apparatus – her executive functions. Another way to say it is that her Central Executive was a bit slow to come on line.

When children go to school, they are faced with normative expectations. In most middle schools, that means study and self-discipline. Carrie had breezed through elementary school because of her native smarts, but buckling down to study was new to her and she was unprepared.

A lot of kids are diagnosed with ADD in Middle School or High School for this reason. They haven't cultivated the self-discipline necessary for the academic challenge. I have met college students, graduate students and medical students who have the same problem. To apply themselves in a new and rigorous way is something for which they are not prepared. Their Central Executive isn't yet strong enough for the new challenges they face.

Most children are diagnosed with ADD when they are young and have just begun elementary school. These are the normative expectations they face: they have to sit still and listen; they have to pay attention to the teacher; they shouldn't bother other children; they have to follow the rules that are new and unfamiliar. They aren't ready for the challenge. They can't sit still or listen, they bother other kids and they don't pay attention. They may be six, seven or eight, but they are as active as five-year-olds.

Children may be smart and well-adjusted but not quite ready for school. They are immature, but the proper term is *dysmature*. They are mature, cognitively -- smart enough to master the 3Rs. They are mature socially, when they aren't in class. Their motor development has matured nicely, perhaps better than most kids. But their capacity for self-control, their Central Executive, isn't quite so mature. Give the child a year, or two, or three, and she will catch up. The self-control systems in her brain were slow to develop but they will.

> Little Timmy, for example, was 7 years old, a healthy, happy boy with a lot of energy. He was smart, ahead of a lot of kids in his second grade, but he couldn't sit still. He would disturb other children and blurt out

answers when it wasn't his turn. He was diagnosed with ADD because he scored 16 on this venerable instrument, developed in the 1960's by Keith Conners, a psychologist and an old friend:

Connor's Abbreviated Rating Scale is shown below, a total of more than 15 is suggestive of ADD/ADHD:

Name:	Not at all (0)	Just a little (1)	Pretty much (2)	Very much (3)
RESTLESS AND OVERACTIVE				
EXCITABLE, IMPULSIVE				
DISTURBS OTHER CHILDREN				
FAILS TO FINISH THINGS - SHORT ATTENTION SPAN				
CONSTANTLY FIDGETING				
INATTENTIVE, EASILY DISTRACTED				
DEMANDS MUST BE MET IMMEDIATELY - EASILY FRUSTRATED				
CRIES OFTEN AND EASILY				
MOOD CHANGES QUICKLY AND DRASTICALLY				
TEMPER OUTBURSTS, EXPLOSIVE AND UNPREDICTABLE BEHAVIOUR				
SUBTOTALS:				

The rating scale that pediatricians use now is longer and more refined, but the principle is the same. ADD is diagnosed on the basis of *reported symptoms*. On the Conners scale, 15 or higher is ADD; 10-14 is subclinical ADD. In clinical practice, that's all it takes.

Timmy scored 'pretty much' or 'very much' on the first six items and 'not at all' on the last four. His score was 16 and he was given Ritalin. He took it for a year and a half. He was never inattentive, restless, excitable, impulsive, etc. after that.

Like Carrie, Timmy took Ritalin for a while, and it helped him to overcome a developmental hurdle. They both would probably have overcome the challenge sooner or later without a drug, but Ritalin did no harm and it alleviated the current problem, to everyone's relief. The drug helped them live up to normative expectations.

Most kids diagnosed with ADD have a Central Executive that isn't quite mature.[*] Here is an ADD fact to prove the point: most children who are treated with stimulants for ADD take a drug for 2 or 3 years. There are a lot of reasons why they stop a medication, but the most common reason is that they no longer need it. They grow out of their ADD.

Carrie and Timmy illustrate something one needs to know about brain development, especially the higher cortical systems that regulate cognition. It isn't regular. Development and maturation are not seamless processes. They don't follow a straight line. Not every cognitive or motor function develops at the same rate in every child or falls into place at the right time. Development is irregular in young children, and even less regular around puberty. It's not uncommon for a child's maturity – cognitive, behavioral or emotional – to take a step backwards at the beginning of adolescence. If you've ever told your adolescent son or daughter they were behaving like a two-year-old, you're underscoring the fact.

As a child grows up, his brain develops and functions are gradually *encephalized*. That means that in early childhood

---

[*] This fact has been the source of criticism by the anti-ADD crowd. They claim that we are drugging children to accommodate an education system that expects every child to be the same. Education should be individualized, they say, and they are right, although how they propose to do it is a mystery to me. There are 50 million schoolkids in the USA and 4 million teachers. Universal education is an industrial enterprise of unparalleled dimensions. It relies on the uniformity of normative expectations.

functions are carried out in lower parts of the brain, parts that are older in evolutionary terms, and more stable. With development and maturation, those functions are encephalized, that is, taken over by the cerebral cortex.

The brain's Central Executive finds its seat in the prefrontal cortex but it doesn't get there right away. It develops gradually from lower, subcortical parts of the brain, especially the basal ganglia, a mass of brain structures that reside immediately below the cortex (i.e., subcortical). The BG are like a little brain themselves and can do almost everything the cortex can do. There are many animals (e.g., birds and lower mammals like rats and mice) who don't have much of a cerebral cortex at all. In those animals, the BG are their main control system. They don't do so bad, for birds, mice and rats.

Young children acquire motor control, communication, emotional expression and socialization quite effortlessly because they are virtually instinctive. They are embedded in the limited, structured space of the BG. The basal ganglia are ancient structures, in evolutionary terms, and their functions are kind of automatic. That's why the vast majority of children meet their early developmental milestones on time. If they are bit late in one, they catch up quickly.

Further development and maturation of brain entails the gradual acquisition of important functions by the cerebral cortex, where they can be elaborated in ways that make us smarter than birds and mice. As children grow, their prefrontal cortex gradually comes online. It's not a simple transition or an easy one. New connections have to be made, neural networks have to be upgraded, and efficient communication has to be established from the frontal cortex to every other part of brain. These events don't happen in a regular fashion. They are highly individualized. Because the cerebral cortex is less structured than the BG, it supports behavior that is considered rather than automatic, exploratory rather than rule-bound, adventurous rather than controlled. Brain control systems are moving into a vast new space that is comparatively unstructured and open to countless variations. They make the transition naturally but the processes are influenced by an individual's genetic endowment and also by training and experience.

Brain development is as diverse as people are. New connections are made faster or slower, some networks are upgraded faster than others, and some brain functions come under efficient regulation before others do. The entire process is so tortuous, one wonders why so many school children actually meet normative expectations. They do, I think, because those 4 million schoolteachers work their tails off.

As it happens, the process of encephalization is most intense during early adolescence. It is a time when the cortex finally takes over the most important control functions of brain. The control systems that govern attention, concentration, self-discipline and perseverance are expected to make a giant leap during Middle and High School years and they do, but not in every child at the same time. Carrie was a smart kid and she had all the advantages at home. For her, elementary school was a breeze. But when she finally had to exercise cognitive control and concentrate on her studies, she was ill-equipped for the challenge. The systems hadn't come online yet. They were stuck for a while in that BG > cortex transition.

If you've ever wondered why early adolescence is an unstable time during a child's life, there is a good reason. The brain has to make a giant leap, and some brains hesitate before they do.

6. ACTIVE MINDS

Are you ready for another developmental variation in ADD's big tent?

> Cam was always in motion. He liked to run and jump and tell himself stories as he did. When he walked he had a little hop. When he read – and he loved to read – his foot shook and his leg twitched. In the morning, his bedclothes were always in a tangle.
>
> Cam was 8 years old and smart as could be. He loved building things with his Erector set or scraps of wood and small pieces of junk he found here and there. He laid out elaborate forts in the woods behind the house. He would turn over a rock in the garden and stare at the bugs and worms he found there. He captured a frog and made a habitat out of an old boat he pulled up out of the woods. At the end of the summer, the family returned to the city and Cam went back to school. He hated leaving the country. He cherished the freedom he had there, where his vivid imagination could run free.
>
> In October, his parents got a call from the teacher. *I'm worried about Cam*, she said. *He's such a smart little boy, but he daydreams. And he's so active. Have you ever thought he might be ADD?* Then they brought him to our clinic.

Cam was no more ADD than the man in the moon. He just had a mind that never stopped. He saw a picture of the Vitruvian man on the wall of my office and he said, *That's Leonard-oh daVincey* (rhymes with Quincey), *Isn't it?* Cam wasn't ADD. He was a bright and sensitive boy with a very active mind.

Very smart children with active minds are our fourth ADD phenotype. They are similar to Henry and Carrie and Tim, because their problems are mild and transient, but they are special in their own way. They have a lot of energy. They are easily bored. Schoolwork may be hard for them but only because they are well ahead of their grade and find routine work boring. They are suffused with mental energy and is they can't use it in creative ways they'll let it out somehow.

You could say that an active mind is a personality trait, and it is something that runs in families. You could also say that it's dysmaturation, a problem with self-control. But it's not a problem that the child will grow out of because it's not really a problem at all. It's a gift. What seems like a lot of superfluous motion is a reflection of an active mind. It will likely be harnessed someday. Cam has imagination. He is cultivating the soul of invention.

Let's give him amphetamine and see if we can stamp it out.

What is an active mind? It's not the same as intelligence, ordinarily defined as *the ability to solve complex problems*. Some intelligent minds are quick and agile, others slow and ponderous. Most of us have minds that are agile at some things, usually the things we do all the time, but slow and ponderous on other occasions, like when we're trying to come up with a good excuse.

An active mind is smart and quick and agile. It has unusual, impulsive energy. Its neural connections run fast and in far-flung directions. The connections may not be easy to follow and they may not always make sense, but they go to interesting places and can be unusually inventive.

We usually associate intelligence with the ability to focus. Children with active minds can focus really well when they are absorbed in something; when they are not, their minds range widely across the landscape. During the dull, boring hours that occupy a child's day, active minds wander. They daydream. That, supposedly, is a bad thing, and sometimes it is. In fact, daydreaming is a healthy exercise for the brain. Minds are built to solve problems, to be sure, but they are also built to wander freely.[18]

Active minds tend to wander, but they are also capable of intense focus, what is called *hyperfocus*. That's why such individuals do better in adolescence and adult life, when they find an absorbing occupation. It is why so many children with active minds gravitate to IT or finance, to science, or to the arts, writing and music. It's also why so many people in those fields didn't do so well in school.

Conventional intelligence is goal oriented. An active mind is goal-oriented only some of the time. Goals imply an external event, a reward of some kind. To an active mind, what is going on inside is usually more rewarding. Active minds have so much going on inside, it's easy to get lost in thought. The active minds of children give rise to hours of happy imaginative play and as they grow up, they never lose the gift. You can say that such children are easily distracted, but they are not necessarily distracted by things going on outside, but by their own thoughts.

Too much daydreaming or doing it in the wrong place at the wrong time can have unfortunate consequences. Children with active minds are usually smart, but academic achievement sometimes eludes them. They may to do better on standardized tests because the tests are challenging. Like games, they let the child mobilize her ability to hyperfocus.

Active minds are energetic and adventurous. They often have active bodies attached to them. Little boys run around and little girls dance. That is perfectly natural and a sign of good health. Nevertheless, the combination of distractibility and high activity suggests the diagnosis of ADD, and many children with active minds are so diagnosed. Stimulant drugs like Ritalin and Adderall are prescribed and they may be useful if hyperactivity and short attention span are especially troublesome, but stimulants should be used with care. If they increase mind-focusing at the expense of mind-wandering, it's not so good; when we are forced to treat such children with stimulants, we recommend days off when they don't need the meds. Raising children with an active mind is a special responsibility. Their minds are complex instruments and heavy-handed treatments may blunt their fine points.

Children with active minds are sensitive to events and react energetically. An active mind is alert, quick, agile, venturesome, animated. People with active minds are youthful, lively, dynamic, indefatigable, even vivacious. Much of the time, they drive you crazy.

There is not an epidemic of ADD, but there are a lot of people who have active minds, and more each day. There is a good reason for that, and I explained on an earlier occasion.* Many of the millions of ADDs among us are people whose minds are quick and agile and powerful when they are fully engaged. They can focus for long spans of time but are impatient with things that do not engage them. In ADD World they are supposed to have short attention spans and to be distractible. That is only stating the obvious. The flaw in the theory is that such individuas have long attention spans and are resistant to distraction when they are engaged. *He doesn't have a short attention span. He can sit for hours in front of the computer all night writing another of his silly books.* They are capable of hyperfocus, which was never something we could say about an MBD child.

If we understood the psychology of an active mind, it would go a long way towards explaining the so-called ADD epidemic. Having lived among this tribe for many years and meeting many more in our clinic, I have an inkling of what their psychology might be.

---

* See <u>Angry, Controlling Children</u>, chapter 16.

THEY ARE HIGH-ENERGY MACHINES.

This is the nexus of the problem, insofar as you can call it a problem. Some people just burn more energy in their heads. Figuratively speaking, of course. Mental energy is like physical energy; some of us have a lot, some not so much and most of us about average. If ADD people are high-energy types, then why to they respond to the energizing amphetamines? The answer to questions like this should keep you reading.

THEY ARE IMPATIENT WITH EVENTS THAT DO NOT ENGAGE THEM. WHEN THEY ARE ABSORBED, THEY CAN FOCUS FOR LONG PERIODS OF TIME.

Everyone is like this but active minds take it to a higher level. Their minds occupy a broader bandwidth. An average mind ranges from -10 (distractible) to +10 (focused), the range of an active mind is from -50 to +50. The lows are lower and the highs are higher.

These traits are more problematic in children, whom we expect to occupy a rather narrow bandwidth. Their lives are circumscribed with rules for hygiene, eating, sleeping, getting along and going to school; the same rules, in fact, that their parents learned from their parents. The behavior we expect of a child is exactly what is expected of every other child in the world.

Adults with active minds usually have made a series of choices to accommodate their wide bandwidth. They are able to avoid things that make them impatient and they can actually make a living by immersing themselves in something that is suitably stimulating. Children, however, are confined and usually with good reason; even smart kids don't always have good judgment. I don't recommend child-rearing absent rules for politeness, hygiene, eating and sleeping, going to school and getting along, but children with active minds don't much like rules.

You will be tempted to reason with the child, but remember, every child needs to learn the finality of *Because I said so*.

THEY ARE UNUSUALLY CONFIDENT; THEY KNOW WHAT THEY LIKE

Active minds tend to be self-centered, but not in an egotistical way.[†] They enjoy being themselves. They can find happiness with their own devices. They find it natural to cultivate their individuality, just as at other times and in other cultures the priority would be fitting in. They like themselves and the way they are.

There is a long tradition that raising children is to teach them sacrifice, discipline and self-control. It was appropriate to a world that was harsh and potentially dangerous. The modern tradition is that children must be allowed to cultivate their individuality. It is a good method in a world that is safe and wildly generous, and where advantaged children have unlimited opportunities. But if you teach a child that the world is wide-open, don't be surprised if she takes you at your word and behaves accordingly.

THEY ARE UNUSUALLY CONFIDENT; THEY TAKE ON MORE THAN THEY OUGHT TO

Adults with active minds like to cultivate their individuality and freedom. They bristle under confinement, which is why so few of them thrive in a bureaucratic, corporate environment. They don't like process and rules. They are confident in their own judgments and are impatient with what they deem unnecessary obstacles.

Because they are smart and energetic, people with active minds are often successful. Because of their wide mental bandwidth, they may spread themselves too thin. This was Marcia's problem; we shall meet her later on.

TOO MUCH ENERGY MAY NOT BE ENOUGH

This is more likely to be a problem among adults, whose lives, you may have noticed, can be enervating, especially because

---

[†] The difference between being an *egoist* and an *egotist*.

active minds have the bad habit of spreading themselves too thin. One's attentional resources are finite. They may not be equal to a life that is so full and rich.

THEY TEND TO BE IMPATIENT

One problem with a quick and agile mind is impatience with slow and ponderous processes. Amphetamines tend to make things seem less slow and ponderous.

An 'active mind' isn't a recognized category in psychology or psychiatry. There isn't a category for people who are alert, quick, agile, venturesome, animated, youthful, lively, dynamic, indefatigable and vivacious. There is a category for people who are high-energy, impatient, injudicious and imprudent, and one of them is ADD. But they are usually the same people. Whether their condition is pathological or not depends on the expectations you have of them. Whether they fit in or not. Whether we like them or find them annoying. Whether their IPO crashes or soars.

The trouble that a child may make for his teachers or parents Is sometimes a reflection of his strengths and not his defects. Such children need to know that their minds are special and capable of great things. 'Great things' may be a bit strong, but many, if not most, of the great figures in history were troublesome students and disappointments to their parents. Adjusting to normative expectations takes time for a child whose mind is accustomed to visiting distant worlds and inventing fantastical characters. An energetic mind is a great gift, but a lot of growing up is needed to bring it under social control.

Here are couple of facts that support my argument:

- If ADD is a form of brain dysfunction, we should be concerned by the fact that half of the schoolchildren with diagnosable ADD are not taking medications at all.

They must be doomed to lives of perpetual dysfunction. Do you believe that?

- Studies of children on stimulant drugs always indicate that they are mostly smart, healthy children from advantaged households. In contrast, *every other cognitive, behavior or emotional disorder in childhood* is concentrated in children in poor health, with learning disabilities and from disadvantaged or dysfunctional families. The present understanding of ADD puts it at variance with every other childhood disorder.

7. WHAT, IF ANYTHING, IS ADD?

What is ADD? The manual defines it with precision. In practice, it is many different things.

In Martin it is a neurodevelopmental disorder caused by injury to his brain. He has what used to be called minimal brain damage. Felix had a similar condition but not nearly so severe, and he didn't have overt signs of neurological impairment. He had what was once called minimal brain dysfunction. Both had a condition that remained troublesome all their lives. In the many countries of the world where the prevalence of ADD is 1 or 2%, the patients are like Martin and Felix.

In the USA, the prevalence of ADD is 5 or 10% or maybe 15%. It's because kids like Henry, Carrie, Timmy and even Cam are diagnosed with ADD. But they don't have a neurodevelopmental disorder. In Henry and his father, what we call ADD is a personality trait. In Carrie and Timmy, it is a transient blip in brain development. Cam's teachers thought he might be ADD, but he was easily bored because he had an active, unfettered mind.

In Felix, we meet the prototype of ADD. He is the one researchers like, because he fits the criteria and has a persistent condition. Remember, Felix was seven when his mother complained that he was overactive, restless and distractible. He had always been active, even as a baby, and was a restless sleeper. He was a good kid but he got in trouble at school for bothering the other children. He couldn't sit still. His pediatrician gave him Ritalin, and when he was in High School, he took Adderall. When he was 18, he aged out of the pediatric practice and was followed in our clinic.

After High School, Felix worked for a while and didn't take Adderall. He went back on it when he went to community college. He didn't finish because he was also working two jobs and then he became assistant manager at MacDonald's. He had to continue taking Adderall, even when he wasn't working, because he tended to get speeding tickets when he was off it. He went back to school, got a degree, and gradually rose to regional manager. He married and had two children. Both of them were having problems at school and so Felix brought them back to me. I hadn't seen him for years. He had been getting Adderall from his primary care doc.

Felix' story underscores the fact that yes, Virginia, there is ADD as the DSM defines it, and not every such patient has signs of a neurological insult. They are the ADD kids who grow up to be adult ADDs. Don't listen to the people who say that ADD is a myth.

Felix is a prototype, but kids like Felix are only a small proportion of the patients diagnosed with ADD. My goal is wider and more inclusive. I want to explain ADD in all its forms and variants.

 What is ADD? *It is one of those mental conditions that exists in severe form in a small number of people while mild forms are very common.*   ADD resembles a lot of other mental conditions, such as anxiety, depression, OCD; severe, disabling forms are not common, but a lot of people are OC or have spells of anxiety or depression.

ADD is a disabling mental *disorder* in about 1 or 2% of children and perhaps 1% of adults. ADD symptoms are a *problem* for ten times as many children and adults. The fact that both groups respond to stimulant drugs doesn't mean they are the same.

ADD exists in severe form in a small number of people while mild forms are very common. Many medical conditions, if not most, are like that; arthritis, hypertension, low back pain, COVID, and even some cancers. Arthritis is a good example. Subclinical arthritis means you don't have to see a rheumatologist or take an immunomodulator. But after a day in the garden, your joints are stiff and you wish you had taken an Ibuprofen the night before. For those many people with ADD symptoms, Adderall is the equivalent of Advil.

ADD, as it stands in 2023, is not precise at all. It is an umbrella term that covers a large number of people, most of whose problems are related to other conditions or nocuous life circumstances.

ADD and all its forms and variants have something in common. They all represent a failure, or a weakness, in a person's ability to regulate his or her cognitive, behavioral or emotional resources. Such weaknesses, or failures, are astonishingly common. They may arise at any age. They may be transient or persistent, mild or severe, disabling or not. The source of the problem resides in the brain regions that participate in self-regulation: that prefrontal cortex (under your palm, remember?) and its Central Executive.

THE BRAIN'S CENTRAL EXECUTIVE

The prefrontal cortex and its connections are the brain's regulatory apparatus. It is responsible for almost every aspect of self-regulation, from basic functions like heart rate and blood pressure on up to higher functions like concentration and self-control. It is the seat the executive functions, whence the terms, Central Executive and executive dysfunction. The executive functions include planning, motivation, perseverance, initiative, multitasking, problem-solving, self-correction and flexibility, that is, changing one's behavior in light of changing events. Sustained and selective attention are also executive functions. The Central Executive governs one's ability to adjust to the requirements of a situation, behaviorally, emotionally and cognitively. It presides over ability to learn from mistakes, to respond appropriately to rewards and punishment and to defer gratification. The regulatory functions underlie how we learn, how we do things, how we respond to intrusions and how well we can direct our endeavors. They are functions crucial to mature adult life. They are functions that ADDs find it hard to master.*

So, Felix had a weak Central Executive, and the weakness was persistent. It wasn't the consequence of brain damage but was probably an inherited problem. His mother's brother was a notorious layabout. In Martin's case, the Central Executive was weak to begin with (his father was ADD) and it was damaged further during a difficult birth. Felix could compensate for his weaknesses, but he remained a patient. Martin was never able to overcome his disability.

Carrie and Tim suffered, for a while, from a transient delay in prefrontal development. Henry and Cam had a Central Executive that was strong and effective in some circumstances and weak in others.

The Central Executive resides in the prefrontal cortex but many other brain regions are also part of it. Its main connections are to a few cortical and subcortical regions but it touches virtually every part of brain. The Central Executive is not a little guy in a corner office behind your eyebrows. It is a complex system of neural networks that connect a few key regions, and thence to the rest of brain.[19] The anatomy of the Central Executive is complicated, and so is the way it behaves.

An effective Central Executive directs behavior in the direction of appropriateness and utility. In its absence, behavior is random or idiosyncratic. An illustration is patients with frontal lobe injuries. They are *stimulus-bound*. That means, when they see something, they have to touch it, pick it up or knock it over, or play with it. They are unable to inhibit their reaction to anything novel. When I examined Martin, he couldn't keep his hands off my stethoscope and reflex hammer. He tried to put the one into his ears and he banged on his legs with the hammer. Normal children are like that at age 2 or 3. They don't

---

* There is a movement afoot to rename ADD the *Executive Function Disorder*. ADD needs another name like I need another hole in my head. EFD. Hmpf. Better than ADHD, I suppose, but it sounds like BFD.

have much of a Central Executive.

The Central Executive is far reaching; it governs an individual's unique style of thinking, feeling, acting and responding; that is, one's personality. The diversity of human personality is a function of the complexity of the Central Executive, how its networks develop and change throughout life. Its characteristics and behavior are prone to innumerable variations.

Finally, the Central Executive is *vulnerable*. It is vulnerable to trauma, as Kurt Goldstein learned from injured soldiers. Brain damage in infants affects the prefrontal cortex indirectly, by damaging the fiber bundles in the white matter.[†] It is affected by low blood flow, high temperatures, low oxygen and toxins like carbon monoxide. It is weakened by disease and chronic pain, by fatigue or sleep deprivation, idleness or stress, alcohol and other drugs. Considering how complex the brain's regulatory apparatus is, it's a wonder than any of us get it right. In fact, most of us don't, at least all the time.

You'd think that Nature would protect Her precious Central Executive better than She did. Considering its importance, it should be buried deep within the brain, surrounded by layers of fluffy myelin. But, no, She put it there, hanging out in your forehead, just waiting to get bopped. There must be a good reason why the prefrontal cortex is so vulnerable to trauma, low oxygen in blood or vascular insufficiency, illness, fatigue and stress, and someday I may figure out what it is.[20]

Nature gave our Central Executive interesting characteristics:

[†] The white matter is the largest component of the cerebral cortex, beneath the grey matter, where cortical neurons reside. The white matter is a collection of innumerable nerve fibers (axons) that connect the neurons. Since most the fibers arise from or project to the prefrontal cortex, damage to the white matter impairs prefrontal function.

- The system is slow to develop. Full development of the prefrontal cortex is not complete until about age 50.
- The rate at which it develops varies from one individual to another. Development is especially variable during childhood and adolescence.
- Once it is fully developed, the quality of the central executive is not uniform. In some few of us it a Ferrari. For most of us, it's a Ford. In a few, it's a Yugo.
- Individual differences in brain self-regulation account for for much of the success or failure we experience in life.
- The regulatory apparatus is not a privileged space. It is affected by one's personality and emotional stability, education and guidance, family support and social circumstances.
- It is a complex system that is vulnerable to injury and to stresses of many kinds.
- The system tends to grow weaker as we age.

ADD is a diverse condition and the symptoms of ADD are common because they arise from a brain regulatory system that is not quite so stable or uniform as we wish it were.

8. ADD OR ANXIETY?

This is a problem that bedevils pediatricians: *Is it ADD or anxiety?* It is the occasion of not a few referrals to our clinic. After our usual comprehensive in-depth and penetrating evaluation, we answer, *Yes.*

> Lilly was 12 years old. She did very well in school but she had to spend hours on homework. *She gets good grades but she has to work so hard for them*, her mother said. She was a lovely girl, sweet and well-behaved although when I met her I thought she was bit tense. She warmed up a bit during the examination and listened attentively to everything her parents and I were talking about. *She is getting good grades*, her mother said, *But she spends so much time on homework. If a picture or a paper isn't perfect, she tosses it and starts over.*
>
> Lilly was a healthy girl and never a behavior problem. She did tend to worry, though. She was a germaphobe and keenly aware of anyone in her class who sneezed or had the sniffles. She was a bit of hypochondriac, too, and stayed home whenever her stomach acted up, which happened often. But she hated going to the pediatrician because of all the sick people she would encounter. She texted her mother often to report the state of her gastro-intestinal tract.
>
> She was also a perfectionist. Her work had to be perfect before she turned it in. She used highlighters in different colors to mark her notes. She numbered every page. She liked to count, too. When she felt nervous, she would count to six and then back to one, repeatedly, timing her breathing to each repetition. That, she found, was so effective she did it all the time, unless she was worried about something and

forgot. I asked her what was special about the number six; she told me that, to the Hebrews, six was a special number. She knew exactly how many stairs there were to the second floor of her house because she counted them whenever she went up, and counted backwards when she came down.

Lilly was a bit tense but her examination was quite normal. She was cheerful and well-spoken. She was also quite certain that she had ADD. When we tested her, her intelligence was well above average but she did poorly on the Stroop test and made a few impulsive errors on the test of response inhibition, one of the attention tests we give to patients.

Lilly and her mother were determined to try a stimulant, and we knew they would find a doctor who would give her one. So we gave her a test dose of methylphenidate, and sent them off to lunch. They would come back in an hour.

Don't worry so much, I wanted to say. As if it were a choice; some people are born worriers. You can imagine how exhausting it must be. If you ask a worrier, they might say it prepares them for the worst. Some worriers think it prevents bad things from happening. An honest worrier will say, *I can't help it*. Most people who worry a lot don't have a good reason at all. It's what they do.

I won't say that worry is an affliction. Most worriers are sensitive people who really care. They are sweet people who want only the best for people they care about. They like things to be neat and orderly, and there's nothing wrong with that. They are conscientious. They worry about being late. They worry that they may not be doing right, or they worry because *you're* not doing right. They tend to be intelligent people who are all too aware that the world can be a dangerous place.

To some people, worrying is automatic, like a habit. It's not necessarily a bad habit, but like every human foible, it can get out of hand. Worrying a lot is a sign of anxiety, which can interfere with what we want to do and how we would like to be. It is a waste of mental energy. Focusing on fears and apprehensions leaves little room to focus on anything else.

Worry, anxiety, apprehension and fear are universal. We all have had it and will again at some point in the future. Some of us have it all the time. Worry and anxiety, however, are not mental disorders. They are common human experiences. There are disabling forms of anxiety. They are *bona fide* mental disorders and not always easy to treat. They are different in severity, although not in kind, from the worries, fears and anxieties that most of us endure. Not that normal anxiety is a walk in the park. Even childish worries can be hard to live with. Lilly, for example, was a worrier and a lot of things made her anxious. She wasn't disabled by anxiety, but it made her life difficult. It also caused attention problems.

Children are notorious worriers. They worry about being separated from their parents, about spiders and thunderstorms, about ghosts, monsters in the closet and the dwarf who lives under the bed. They may worry about having enough friends, about germs or climate change. A little girl I knew worried that her father was going to die when he left on a business trip. Some kids worry about getting good grades in school or making the travel team. But the common anxieties of childhood are not anxiety disorders and neither are they adumbrations of anxiety disorders to come. They are normal fears and phobias. You may read that anxiety *disorders* are very common in children; some studies estimate they afflict 40% of children. Others report prevalence rates around 10%, but even that number suggests that researchers are classifying normal childhood fears and worries as anxiety disorders. Studies that report the prevalence at 2% are closer to the mark.

Social anxiety and obsessive worry are common childhood problems, perhaps 40% of kids, but most of the time they are comparatively mild problems that abate over time. They may cause difficulties like the problems Lilly was having with schoolwork. They may require a short course of treatment, in therapy or with a medication, but only a small number of those children will grow up to have a disabling mental condition.

This is the message we really send to the pediatrician: *Lilly has anxiety and obsessive worries. She does not have an anxiety disorder. She has mild attention problems which occur in the context of anxiety and an OC disposition. I think we can help her.*

I hear this a lot: *Yes, she gets excellent grades. But she always has to work much harder than anyone else.*

Lilly has a problem with anxiety. Yet she complains of problems with focus and distractibility because schoolwork is inordinately difficult for her. In fact, she met diagnostic criteria for Anxiety and ADD. Does that mean she has two mental disorders? Poor kid.

She has two disorders if you ask the Mechanical Turk. Type in the symptoms: anxiety and inattention. The Turk whirrs and clanks, the mechanical arm reaches into the bin and pulls out a diagnosis: *She has ADD.* But, wait, the Turk is not finished! He pulls out another one: *She has an anxiety disorder.*

Lilly doesn't have two mental disorders. She has two problems, both of which are very common in childhood. (1) She worried too much, in an obsessive way. (2) It was so distracting to her, she had difficulty getting her work done. Lilly had mild attention problems which occurred in the context of anxiety and an OC disposition.

Is there a good reason to understand Lilly's circumstances as problems rather than disorders? It sounds like a distinction without much difference. In fact, the distinction highlights the relatively benign nature of most childhood problems. The child and her parents need to understand that her condition is not severe; if any of her symptoms outlast childhood, they will be mild and well within the wide range of normal. Parents also need to know that whatever treatment is prescribed, it will only be needed for a short period of time. [21]

Lilly is a good example of what energy-hogs anxiety and worry can be. You can imagine how much mental bandwidth the worry habit consumes. Attention is a limited resource that she was wasting on worry. Lilly's obsessive worries and intrusive thoughts sapped her energy and she couldn't do anything else. She was easily distracted from her schoolwork and took too long to get it done. Her mind was so full of worries, she couldn't stop. When she went to bed, she said, she couldn't turn her mind off.

Impaired concentration is one of the symptoms of an anxiety disorder. But it's not only anxiety disorders that interfere with attention and performance, but also the common fears and worries of everyday life. A good illustration is test anxiety, which is extremely common in young people – about 25%, they say. Children with test anxiety are as intelligent as other kids, but they are more likely to do poorly in school, to get lower grades and to repeat a grade. Math anxiety – about 20% of us have math anxiety – is another good example. People with math anxiety perform well below their true ability on math tests.

Attention is a limited resource and if it's devoted to worry there is scarcely enough for anything else. Psychologists have elaborated on this simple explanation. They say there is a *resource allocation mechanism* inside one's head. If they are right, we could say that anxiety forces it to allocate attentional resources to worry. In fact, anxious individuals are more distracted from their work by extraneous events. It's because they have a cognitive bias that colors their perception of ordinary events. They are more likely to perceive ordinary events as threatening. Lilly, for example, was distracted during her homework because all the pencils in her pencil-cup were not perfectly sharp. As dangers so, unsharpened pencils are low on the scale, but it was something that threatened Lilly's equanimity. Anxious individuals are inclined to scan their horizon to make sure no dangers are lurking. Anxious people find it hard to concentrate on a task for fear they will miss one.[22]

That resource allocation mechanism, BTW, is no less than brain's Central Executive and it governs, among other things, what we will attend to, that is, what is allowed to enter our conscious awareness. One's Central Executive consigns mental energy to concentration. It is called *top-down attention*, an act of the will. Another kind of attention is called bottom-up because it arises in lower parts of the brain that process sensation. *Bottom-up attention* is when one responds to an extraneous event. A loud noise in the next room will automatically focus your attention on that room where your cat is in the habit of knocking over the philodendron. The sudden, loud noise is compelling, even if you were engrossed in a good book at the time. Anxious people are bothered by too much bottom-up attention. The most trivial stimulus can seize their attention as if the cat were firing a gun.[23]

Anxious people experience shivers of bottom-up attention that distract their Central Executive from its top-down task. We don't know if the lower parts of their brain are too sensitive or if their Central Executive is too weak. In one study, anxious individuals had more difficulty generating energy in their prefrontal cortex to keep focused on a task when distracting stimuli were presented.[24] That suggests they have a mental weakness similar to what ADD people have.

Lilly made perfect grades but she always had to work much harder than anyone else. When a patient tells you that, it means their attention problems stem from anxiety. That's because mild anxiety decreases the efficiency with which we work. It doesn't necessarily affect the quality of the work and may even improve it, but it's hard to get work done when one is contending with a sluggish Central Executive. That's why Lilly had to work so hard, and why her work was so exhausting.

Fatigue is another common symptom of anxiety. Worriers have a cognitive bias towards perceiving innocent events as threatening. You can imagine how much energy that consumes. Also, what it does to one's biological stress response. Worry generates stress hormones. Over time, hormones like cortisol impair the activity of *mitochondria*, tiny fellows in cells that generate energy.[25] Worry is exhausting.

Does anxiety make you ADD? After all, it affects the same mechanisms that are awry in ADD, and anxious kids often have attention problems. No, *Lilly has mild attention problems which occur in the context of anxiety and an OC disposition.* Sounds like another distinction without much difference, I admit. Psychiatrists finesse the distinction by saying that Lilly has *comorbid* ADD and anxiety; in other words, two mental disorders. Such thinking is what gives us anxiety rates of 40% and four million children on amphetamines. It would also give Lilly prescriptions for Ritalin *and* Lexapro.

Good psychiatrists aren't Mechanical Turks and would understand Lilly to be a smart, healthy girl who needs a bit of help. They would assure Lilly and her parents that her problems were common in children and unlikely to lead to chronic mental illness. Lilly herself knew that she was a worrier and that it was a bad habit. She and her parents didn't know that worry can cause attention problems and that treating her anxiety would fix them.

Nevertheless, Lilly was preoccupied with ADD and wanted to try a stimulant. She did have problems with attention on one of the tests we gave her. I warned her that Ritalin might upset her delicate stomach but she wanted to try anyway. So we gave her a test dose of Ritalin. She came back an hour later; short-acting Ritalin begins to peak after 45 minutes. When she re-took our tests, she made fewer errors on the test of response inhibition, but she made more mistakes on the Stroop test. Her sensitive GI tract was OK but she felt jittery on the drug. Lilly was not impressed, nor her mother, nor me.

Lilly did well after she started seeing a therapist who understood children who were prone to obsessive worry. At some point she may have to try a low dose of an SSRI antidepressant like Lexapro, but I had a feeling that therapy would be all she needed. But for every child like Lilly who did poorly on a stimulant, there is another child with similar problems who does better. We have no way of predicting. That's why we give kids a test dose before we prescribe a stimulant.

Lilly's attention problems were secondary to her anxious, OC disposition. She should do better if her anxiety were treated, and she did. But another child whose primary problem is anxiety might do well on a stimulant. Interesting; as a rule, stimulant drugs make anxious people more anxious. How to explain the fact that so many people with anxiety respond to stimulant drugs?

Here is how I explain it to parents:

> Your child has problems with attention that stem from her anxious, OC disposition. We could treat him with an SSRI. That will improve his anxiety and his attention problems might also get better. Or we could try a stimulant, which will improve his attention and may also help him control his anxiety. Which step should we take first?

Parents are pretty good at recognizing priorities. If the child did well after a stimulant test dose, they might well opt for a stimulant trial. *Doing better at school will make him feel more confident.* Or they might say, *He's doing well enough in school for now, in spite of his attention problems. He needs something for anxiety.*[26]

9. ADD OR OC?

Lilly's anxiety was the consequence of an OC disposition. That doesn't mean that she had obsessive-compulsive disorder. OCD is not a common mental disorder, but at least a third of us have a few OC traits, and Lilly had more than a few. Children are as prone to obsessions and compulsions as they are to anxiety, attention problems and fidgeting. They aren't usually bothersome but may become so if the stars are misaligned.

> Lilly was a picky eater. She only ate one thing at a time and she hated her food to touch on the plate. If someone drank from her cup, she would get up and get a new one. In the restrooms at school she would flush with her feet, she used paper towels to turn on the taps and pushed the doors open with her elbow. She knew exactly how many stairs there were to the second floor of her house because she counted them whenever she went up, and counted backwards when she came down.

I wrote a book about OC, The OCD of Everyday Life. You might find a copy in a rare book store. In the book I suggested that it's not so bad to be OC.* Most OCs are conscientious and good-hearted, when they aren't worried about something. Obsessive worry is the downside of OC, and a lot of OCs worry because they can't focus. Then they read one of those self-help books and decide, I must be ADD. Not a few of our adult ADDs are OCs who are effective but not efficient. It makes them tired and grumpy and then they worry even more. Until a good-hearted physician gives them Adderall, that is. Then they worry that they're not getting enough.

We shall meet a number of OCs in these pages; you probably

---

* There are bad OCs, though. Read about them in another book of mine, Angry Controlling Children.

have encountered more than few yourself. They may be neatniks, obsessive worriers, perfectionists or compulsive exercisers, especially cyclists and body-builders. They are given to odd hobbies and collections. They aren't hoarders but they don't like to throw things away. They may be fastidious, germ-phobic, fussy, superstitious or controlling. Their minds tend to be busy; many have active minds, quick and agile, but slow when they are riven with obsessive concerns. Many seem to be wound up tight. They need everything to be just right; loading the dishwasher correctly is a common preoccupation. The worst is when they worry that something is not right but they don't know what it is. So they check the doors to make sure they are all locked, the stove to make sure it's off and, of course, the dishwasher. I'm sure that *you* never put plastics on the bottom shelf.

A mind thus cluttered is not especially efficient. Intrusive worries are distracting. OCs are also notorious procrastinators. When their productivity suffers accordingly, they decide that they must be ADD. They get hung up on the idea, *I need Adderall*, and the vast, commanding ADD industry is there to oblige.

> Milo was a PhD student in biostatistics at one of the most prestigious programs in the country. He had always excelled at school but now he had a problem: his dissertation. He had done extremely well in an internship at the FDA and another with a pharmaceutical company. He could have his choice of jobs as soon as he finished his degree. His dissertation was a masterful bit of research and the analysis was well within his ability. He had just about got it done but he couldn't get it down on paper. He would stare at his notes while his mind wandered. *I can't keep my focus on the thing. I must be ADD.*

Milo had writer's block, right? Or was it fear of success? Or fear of leaving the womb of subsidized graduate education... I should have recommended therapy, or hypnosis, or a nice vacation. But first I had to address his concerns. He wanted amphetamine.[27]

Milo was a slight young man with big dark eyes that seemed bigger because of his intense manner. He acknowledged that he was a perfectionist – one trait, BTW, that is known to be associated with writer's block. He had seen a counsellor on campus, who must deal with this sort of thing often. The counsellor suggested he might have ADD.[28]

OC IS DISTRACTING

Perfectionism is a form of OC. It's not necessarily bad, especially if one is responsible for vast quantities of important medical data. *Don't let perfect be the enemy of the good* is a familiar expression, but statistical analysis has to be close to perfect. It is a likely place for a conscientious OC to get embroiled in petty details and worry over imperfections. OCs are slow getting things done; prioritizing and winnowing are not in their nature.

OCs have a hyperactive error detector and can be plagued by the feeling that *Something is wrong here.* Normal worriers fret that something bad might happen; obsessive worriers are disquieted because it already has, only they aren't sure what it is. Imagine producing a 300-page dissertation, occupying six months of steady work, and beneath it all there is a lurking worry that *something is wrong here.*

OCs in general and perfectionists in particular are notorious procrastinators. They find a hundred things that have to get done before they can properly attend to the task at hand. When they try to work, intrusive, anxiety-provoking thoughts get in the way. *OMG, how will I ever get this important task done?* Then, worrying that one may have intrusive, anxiety-provoking thoughts becomes an intrusive, anxiety-provoking thought. To avoid this vicious circle they procrastinate.

I have had the privilege to work with more than one perfectionist. One of my colleagues was so obsessive he could barely complete his daily notes, let alone a patient report. If he ever completed one, it might be a marvel of clarity and clinical analysis. Or it might be a jumble of disconnected facts. You never knew what you were going to get. Whichever, it took a long time to get it and most of the time you got nothing at all. He would leave his notes unfinished. There was always something he had to add and he would when he got around to it. He told me once, *When I take twice my usual dose of dextro-amphetamine I do better keeping up with my notes.*

OCs LIKE STIMULANT DRUGS

OCs *like* ADD. There is something about ADD that appeals to them: amphetamines. Low doses of stimulants help with focus and distractibility, speed up slow processing speed, help with initiation, perseverance and productivity. They make you feel good and more energetic. Stimulants are safe drugs, as long as one keeps to low doses, and they are usually more effective than any of the other stimulants out there: caffeine, nicotine, alcohol, betel-nut, ginseng, qat and high doses of sugar. Amphetamines are about a stimulating as a good, strong physical work-out but they don't make you sweat.

Stimulants appeal to different kinds of people. Patients with manic-depression have notable problems with attention and they like to take stimulants. It's not a good idea because stimulants can make them manic. Some of them don't mind because they like being manic. Sociopaths like stimulants because they can sell them. Druggies like to grind them up and snort them, that is, if they can't find crack cocaine or crystal meth. I have met more than one idle layabout who insisted he needed Adderall because he couldn't focus. All he did all day was lie on the couch and watch TV. Nothing is worse than a short attention span, I suppose, when one is watching TV.[†]

[†] Stimulants are performance-enhancing drugs. If you're not into anything in the way of performance, do you really need a stimulant?

There are special risks, however, to giving stimulants to OCs. When one takes a stimulant, it confers a boost of energy and a bit more focus and concentration. The drug does that whether one is ADD or not, and it can do it even if one's attention problems are caused by anxiety, obsessive ruminating, chronic hypomania or daily doses of cannabis. *It's the only thing that helps me go to sleep,* the patient says, referring to cannabis. He needs cannabis to sleep because he's taking so much amphetamine. He needs a stimulant because he uses so much cannabis.

One problem is that the effects of stimulants are noticeable; they are 'on-off' drugs. That means the patient experiences the positive effects of the drug when it is acting and then the negative effects of the drug wearing off. The danger of giving a stimulant to an OC is that the drug is *conditioning* him to monitor his internal state. It is the problem of obsessive self-monitoring. The patient was already prone to ruminating over perceived deficits; the stimulant effect gives him one more thing to obsess over. He is led to brood over the effects of drug withdrawal: *This ADD is killing me. I don't have enough Adderall!* He tells his doctor just that and gets a higher dose to take.

Which leads to a second problem. Small doses of stimulants are effective at improving cognitive performance. Higher doses have the opposite effect. Taking a higher dose, the patient experiences more cognitive lapses than he had before he started. His reaction? *I don't have enough Adderall.* Finally, he is taking enough amphetamines to fuel a trucker driving from Halifax to Tijuana and he still wants more. At this point his family doc gets nervous and sends the fellow to our clinic. After our usual evaluation, we tell the patient that he is on an amphetamine treadmill, that his problem is OC not ADD, and that he needs to get off the stuff. He usually becomes quite irate and looks for another psychiatrist.

It is odd practice to treat obsessions with drugs that simply increase the patient's proneness to obsess, or to treat a cognitive disorder with a drug that can impair one's cognition, but ADD World wouldn't thrive as it does if it didn't countenance just that sort of thing. Physicians who make their patients worse are held in high esteem as long as they make them feel better for a while, and as long as they prescribe a higher dose next time.

ADD TRAITS AND OC TRAITS

About half of the children who are evaluated at our clinics for ADD have OC traits. More than half of our adult patients who think they are ADD are OCs. ADD and OC are both constellations of personality and cognitive traits that cluster, in severe forms, in a relatively small number of people. Mild forms of ADD and OC occur in many more people and meld into the common, day-to-day weaknesses that everybody has.

ADD and OC are opposites with only superficial similarity. ADD is a flaccid attentional muscle and OC is an attentional muscle that has been exercised too much. At the level of elementary neurobiology, ADD is a brain problem with central regulation; that is, not enough.[29] OC is also a problem with brain regulation, but *too much*. On a cognitive level, ADDs are distracted by events going on in the outside world. OCs are distracted by events going on inside their heads. On a behavioral level, ADD's tend to be disinhibited, or wide-open. OC's are up-tight. ADD's are resilient; bad experiences hurt for a while, then roll off their backs. OCs tend to brood. OCs never forget; ADDs forget all the time. On an interactional level, ADDs are stimulating but exhausting. OCs are secure and predictable but boring.

I asked Milo if he had ever taken a stimulant before and he had, when he was in college, but he got it from friends and only used it to stay up and study. I convinced him that he would do better on an SSRI, and he did. He would have done equally well with a counsellor who knew his problem wasn't ADD.

PART TWO

ADD IN ADULTS

My colleagues and I first wrote about ADD adults in 1985.[29] The DSM at the time called it 'Attention Deficit Disorder, Residual Type.' We studied a group of adults who met the criteria and found they had little in common and probably didn't represent a 'distinct clinical entity.'

Adults with ADD symptoms are even more diverse than ADD children. Nevertheless, they fall into the same categories. Some are like Martin and Felix -- the real thing: neurodevelopmental disorders that persist into adult life.

Many more are like Tim and Carrie, who had transient ADD symptoms that self-corrected as they matured. They had difficulty adjusting to new academic challenges. Many adults with ADD symptoms find themselves facing challenges for which they are unprepared.

Lilly and Milo had ADD symptoms that arose as a consequence of another mental problem. So, too, with many adults.

We shall meet a number of adults with ADD and with ADD symptoms. They introduce us to the wider range of problems that cause symptoms that look like ADD.

10. WHAT, IF ANYTHING, IS ADULT ADD?

Martin and Felix were ADD children who grew up to be ADD adults. Not every case, though, is so straightforward.

> Kim was a lively child, good at school and she was a swimmer in High School. She was also a bit of mischief when she was young. She was an obedient daughter but she didn't really like rules. As a teenager, she regarded rules as challenges, to break them without her parents finding out. Every once in while she'd get into trouble, but she'd make up for it and carry on. She graduated with good grades and went to our local college.
>
> In college there were few rules but the lack of challenge didn't deter her adventuresome spirit. It took her 10 years and three colleges to get a degree. In between, she worked, made good money and lived independently. She married before she finally graduated and had her first baby while she worked on her Masters. Then she got a promotion, a second baby, a better job and another promotion.
>
> She was always a lively spirited woman, but she was given to moods. She was in therapy a couple of times and a doctor gave her Prozac once. She took it and it helped for a while. Then, when she was in her third college, someone suggested she might be ADD. She has been taking Adderall, now, for ten years.

ADD – real ADD – comes in all sizes and shapes. Like Henry, Kim had those personality traits we talked about. They weren't disabling although she did do risky things and her academic career fell off the tracks for a while. She might have done better if she had been diagnosed earlier but judging from her career, husband and beautiful children, she did pretty well. Laboring in the vineyards for seven years prepared her well. She made a fortuitous career choice and was highly successful.

Kim was never identified as an ADD when she was in school because she was able to compensate. She lived a structured family life and had so many positive attributes. In college, she had less structure and the academic demands were greater. She hit a wall and decided to leave school. Yet she spent her next few years working, supporting herself and, well, having fun. Her high energy and positive disposition served her well. Then she outgrew that stage of her life.

It took a few years of maturation, a solid relationship, and a baby before she got serious. She did well at college #3. Then she discovered she had been ADD all along. She takes Adderall now, a low dose but just about every day.

When she's at work, at home, keeping up with three little kids and a husband who is off somewhere on one of his projects, she takes Adderall every day. When she doesn't, she feels scattered and ineffective. It isn't necessarily a withdrawal reaction. It's like a flashback to the bad old days when she felt scattered, when she was effective but not efficient.

The diagnostic criteria require symptoms to have been present before age 12. Kim didn't have symptoms then. Neither did Jennifer.

> Jennifer was 55. She worked in Inventory Control at one of our nearby industrial plants. She was healthy, a bit heavy perhaps, and she had always been active. She never married and her long-term boyfriend had died a few years back. She had no children but worked as a volunteer at the Animal Shelter and went on a church mission every year. She came to the clinic because she was having memory problems. She did well at work and was promoted to supervisor in her

department. Now she had trouble keeping up with all her responsibilities, was forgetful and felt scattered.

Jennifer was lively and vivacious. She had never been prone to anxiety or moods and this was her first visit to a psychiatrist. When we tested her, her memory was fine. She didn't have any dementia risk factors. But she did poorly in several tests of attention.

Jennifer had done OK in school but she left college after a year. Testing showed that she was smart enough to have done welll in college but she admitted that she could never attend to lectures because her mind would wander.

We gave Jennifer a test dose of Ritalin and she did very well. She felt more organized and her test scores improved.

One problem with adult ADD is that symptoms may not have been overt before the patient was 12 years old, as the diagnostic criteria require. Smart kids, especially smart girls, tend to do OK in school even if they are ADD. When Kim and Jennifer were children, their ADD was 'subclinical' or 'latent'. Later in life they encountered challenges that evoked ADD symptoms. At that point, the symptoms became clinical and the disorder was overt. Stimulant drug treatment was appropriate, and effective. Were they *real* ADDs?

We routinely ask patients, Were you ever diagnosed with ADD or a learning disability in school? Patients like Kim and Jennifer respond like this:

> *Back then nobody knew about ADD.*
> *My parents never had me evaluated.*
> *I was never a very good student.*
> *I always had to work harder than everybody else.*

Sounds like what Lilly's mother told me: *She is getting good grades, but she spends so much time on homework.* How to know an ADD adult is really ADD?

It's easier to give patients a ten-item rating scale, add up the numbers and pronounce the diagnosis if they score over 15. It erases the need for reflection and critical judgment. A careful history is more challenging.

This is another ADD criterion that neither Kim nor Jennifer met: "The presence of significant impairment in at least two major settings of the person's life." Examples are marital conflict, getting fired or going bust because of impulsive spending. Martin and Felix met that criterion, but most adult ADD patients don't.

I am not suggesting the criteria be changed, only that there is vast number of mild ADDs out there, and most are like Kim and Jennifer and Henry's father. *ADD exists in severe form in a small number of people while mild forms are very common.* The boundary between real ADDs and people with ADD symptoms is blurry sometimes.

And so it will remain. It has to do with that Central Executive of ours. It's not digital. It's not either-or, effective or ineffective. It's usually somewhere in between, effective sometimes and a fumbler at others; competent in some but not circumstances; good at some things but not everything. The Central Executive is decidedly analog. Sometimes it is weak from the start and remains so.[30] In adults with ADD symptoms, the Central Executive has gone awry because something is interfering, like stress or anxiety, or it isn't strong enough to surmount a new challenge. The brain's regulatory apparatus is not a complex system like an airliner or a nuclear submarine that has to work perfectly every time, all the time. It's more like a muscle, another biological structure that is strong or weak, ready or not, tired out or sometimes it just hurts.

The fuzzy boundary between real ADD and ADD symptoms

creates problems for clinicians, even those endowed with critical judgment and the time to take a good clinical history. It is also a porous boundary, and that accounts for the fact that in 2014, for the first time, more stimulant prescriptions were written for adults than for children. Adult ADD seems to be everywhere. We are told, in medical papers, that the prevalence rate of adult ADD is around 2.5%. However, when ADD is defined 'broadly' the rate goes up to 16.4% -- one in eight Americans. A national survey in 2016 found that about 4.5% of US adults (11 million) used prescription stimulants 'appropriately' in the preceding year. The numbers are higher now, but in 2016 they were higher than during three previous, unlamented amphetamine epidemics in Japan and Sweden after the Second World War and in the USA during the 60s.[31]

The numbers are astonishing and suggest that, under the guise of ADD, normal, healthy people are using amphetamines to alleviate everyday mental or physical fatigue. Some people like amphetamines for a little boost now and then, or every day. Some of them are convinced, *I'm ADD and I can't do without Adderall.* Most of them, however, are like Kim and Jennifer and Henry, Sr. They have mild symptoms that are only disabling when they are confronted with challenges they are unprepared for.

As it happens, real ADDs as well as patients like Kim and Jennifer can be treated successfully with psychostimulants. Successful treatment means alleviation of patients' problems without side effects, habituation or addiction.

But are they *real* ADD's? There is a category in the ICD* that fits them better: *R41.840 Attention and concentration deficit.* But it's an R code, not a diagnosis, and insurance won't pay for an R code.

---

* The International Classification of Diseases, published by the World Health Organization, and used by third-party payers to justify reimbursement.

11. THE STIMULANT HABIT

Elspeth was 21 years old, a student at an elite college in New York. Her GPA at East Chapel Hill High School was 6.0 and she had straight As in college. She was a lovely young lady, well-spoken but serious and a bit intense. She had been treated for ADD since High School and was still taking 20 mg of Adderall twice a day. She had aged out with her pediatrician and had to find a new prescriber. When she came to us, she was annoyed that we had to do a full evaluation. *Its all been done*, she said. *All I need is a prescription*. For adolescents and young adults, the evaluation usually entails a urine drug screen for illicit drugs.

Elspeth's examination was perfectly normal and she did very well when she was tested. The only test that gave her a bit of trouble was the Stroop test; she got every response right but her processing speed was slow. Her urine drug screen was positive for amphetamine (Adderall) but also for cannabis and benzodiazepines.

She told me that she smoked weed at the end of the day to help her sleep. She got the Xanax from a friend but only took it occasionally. I told her that she was in the unenviable position of using uppers in the morning and downers at night. I don't make a fuss over occasional marijuana, but she was using it medicinally, and that suggested something else was wrong. I wasn't about to help her play that game.

That led to a rather long and dreary argument about drug laws and how I was wrong to suggest she was hurting herself. She was healthy and happy and had a boyfriend. She had just done a fabulous internship in California and when she graduated, they wanted her to come back. Now, she felt like talking. I guess her Adderall was kicking in.

The boyfriend, it turned out, was a schoolmate and it was he who gave her Xanax. They did cocaine together, too; he must have been the campus dealer. Cocaine, she said, was just for parties, or else she liked MDMA (Ecstasy). Ketamine was OK but she didn't use opioids very often because she liked them too much. She assured me that she didn't do heroin very often and was always safe when she injected it.

Elspeth had everything. She came from a good family; her father was an orthopedist and her mother was an internist. She had two sisters who were almost as smart as she was, but not quite so adventurous. She went to the best college and had no student debt. She was healthy, attractive and very smart. She wasn't going to California when she graduated, but to Peru, where she would study the role of women in the Andean labor movement. It was work of seminal importance, she told me, and she would get a Fulbright.

'Adventurous' is a word she used to describe herself and it seemed right to a 21-year-old. 'Oblivious' is the word that occurred to me. Risk, to Elspeth, was something to enjoy, not avoid. It was something she liked to live with, ensconced as she always had been in safe, giving environments. Danger was not in her vocabulary.

Elspeth had an unusually active mind, which in most circumstances would be reward enough. But she had an unusual desire to change its normal parameters with mind-altering drugs. She had been using cannabis and borrowing her mother's Ativan before she ever thought of taking a stimulant. When she got a few Adderalls from a friend she enjoyed the mild euphoria, alertness, energy and ability to get a whole lot done. It took a bit of doing to convince her pediatrician that she was ADD, but she did. So, she took Adderall regularly from tenth grade on. In college, her drug use grew more inclusive, but Adderall was her foundation drug. It kept her alert for serious business, like lectures, seminars and writing papers. She also found it was good for reversing the fatigue she experienced after a weekend of partying. Too much cannabis or heroin the night before made it hard to get up. She would set her alarm a half-hour early and take an Adderall. She would sleep until the drug woke her up.*

There are many different reasons why people use illicit drugs and many more reasons why they get addicted, but this chapter is about a special case. It's not an uncommon one. In our wealthy, healthy and unusually advantaged society, people can avail themselves of an extraordinary number of mind-altering substances and a lot of them do. The term for it is 'recreational drug use' but the term isn't universally applicable. People often use drugs like cannabis and amphetamine with functional rather than hedonic intent; to alleviate stress, to enhance energy, to feel more alert, etc. We should call it *purposeful* or *functional* use. The number of such users is far higher than that of compulsive, destructive drug users, whom we know as addicts. Functional drug users take drugs, not to get high but for their positive effects, like alertness and freedom from fatigue. Using drugs in that way can turn into a habit.

Elspeth's habit is interesting. She has an active mind that enjoys expanding its boundaries. She wants to broaden her range of experience. She is a controlling young woman and likes to control her mental state. She is impatient. She is used to things coming easily and she can use drugs intelligently to achieve the mental state she wants. She is smart. She thinks she knows how to take risks, when to do it and with whom. In that

---

* If only she has been born twenty years later. In 2020 a form of Ritalin was introduced that didn't start to work until 10 hours after it had been ingested. The drug isn't absorbed until it reaches the colon. It is a wake-up pill for ADD children and only costs $500 per month. You can't make these things up.

context, warning her about the dangers of unsupervised drug use, which include cerebral hemorrhage, panic attacks, infertility, brain damage, psychosis and sudden death, doesn't have an impact.

With no small measure of good luck, Elspeth survived her adventures in the drug world. I saw her ten years later when she was visiting her parents. She was a tenure-track professor at a college in the Northeast and her boyfriend was an investment banker. At some point they would marry because she wanted to have a baby. She honored me with a visit in spite of our earlier disagreements because she wanted my ideas about drugs and pregnancy. Her poly-drug use was history but she still smoked cannabis at night and took Adderall in the morning. Cannabis helped her sleep and Adderall made her more productive. She was happy and healthy, she told me. She didn't think the drugs would affect the fetus, but she knew I would always give her a good argument and she wanted my opinion.

She knew how to access the medical literature on the internet, but she wasn't happy with what she found there. Taking methylphenidate or amphetamine may have adverse effects on a pregnancy but the risk of fetal malformation is very low and the amounts of medication excreted in breast milk are very small. But are they really safe? The FDA evades the question; the drugs are pregnancy category C, with "insufficient information to confirm either harm or lack of harm".[32] Neither stimulants nor cannabis are overtly teratogenic; they don't cause major fetal malformations. Both can affect fetal growth. If they affect brain development, the effects are subtle. The drug effects are difficult to separate from the other problems that cannabis and stimulant users have. Users tend to be young mothers, less well-educated and often have inadequate prenatal care. They often use tobacco, alcohol, and other drugs.[33] It is hard to know the fetal effects of a drug when the effects are small and when mothers suffer many other disadvantages.

No one knows the fetal effects of cannabis + amphetamine. Nevertheless, cannabis and psychostimulants are the commonest drugs consumed by pregnant women in the US and other developed countries. The rate of drug use is increasing, so we shall get better answers about their safety in a few years.

What I told Elspeth is right out of the book: one can't assume that it is safe to use cannabis or psychostimulants during pregnancy. The risk to the fetus is small but not negligible. No one knows the fetal effects of cannabis + amphetamine. Fetal brain development is a complex process and we don't know if the drugs interfere with optimal development in subtle ways. Anyway, we don't share cannabis or amphetamine with little babies; why give them to a fetus?[34]

I asked her what happened when she didn't smoke cannabis at night. She said she couldn't sleep. What happened if she didn't take Adderall? *I can hardly get out of bed. I can't get anything done.* What happened if she didn't take either? She never tried.

You can't say that Elspeth was addicted, because that implies self-destructive drug use. She could have taken better care of herself, to say the least, but in spite of her habits she was healthy and successful and likely to remain so. She was, however, dependent on the drugs. She cringed when I compared her to a smoker who is addicted to nicotine. *Smoking is bad for your health,* she would say, *But there is no danger to low doses of cannabis or stimulants.* She conceded that she was dependent. Cannabis and Adderall had become habits that she found no reason to break. She deemed them *functional habits*.

We know all about stimulant addiction. It is probably the most destructive of all addictions; at least it was until fentanyl came along. Addiction to meth and other stimulants is still with us in enormous numbers. The Adderall explosion, however, has introduced a new problem, even if we don't know how problematic it is. Habitual, functional use is different; it is not immediately or overtly destructive. Habitual, functional use means the individual uses amphetamine on a regular basis to improve an important function and does so without apparent ill effects. The patient has done so for so long, it is hard to know whether he still needs the drug. When he stops using, he experiences a decline in alertness, attention, energy and motivation. That only proves that he was dependent on the drug, not that he needed it in the first place.

Here is a common scenario: a young man comes to the clinic. He is 30 years old and has been taking stimulants since middle school. Now he is on 15 mg of long-acting Dexedrine, the same dose for several years. When he doesn't take the drug, he feels tired and inattentive. The assumption is that he has ADD and is a stimulant responder. He gets a new prescription. Are we treating persistent ADD or are we feeding a stimulant habit?

In Elspeth's case, we know that she was never ADD. She started using Adderall in the context of adolescent poly-drug abuse. She was an habitual user with no good reason for taking the drug in the first place. In the young man's case, he has always taken a moderate dose and always under medical supervision. He never did drugs and hardly ever drinks. But there is no way to know if his initial treatment in middle school was for a very good reason. All we know is that he is dependent on the drug now.

The only way to know whether the fellow really needs Dexedrine is to stop the drug for a while. It takes at least two weeks to get over the effects of stimulant withdrawal and establish a baseline. What we would do in the clinic is to test him when he was finally over his withdrawal reaction, and then test him after a test dose in the clinic.

Why go through all the trouble? Elspeth would say, *If you can't find ill effects of stimulants on a fetus, what makes you think low doses have bad effects on adults?* I would tell her to read on. Are there ill effects to functional stimulant use? We shall get to that soon enough.

11. OBSESSIVE SELF-MONITORING

Something else happened when Elspeth starting using drugs, more interesting than just a bad habit. She changed how she thought about herself. Using short-acting drugs as she did in High School – cannabis, Adderall, her mother's Xanax – she experienced herself on-and-off the drugs, repeatedly, sometimes more than once a day. So doing, she learned to monitor her mental state. She also learned that she could manipulate it at will. During her formative adolescent years, she developed an obsession with her mental state and a compulsion to control it.

States of mind are always in flux, especially mood states, energy states and the state of one's cognitive apparatus. One is cheerful or glum, alert or dull, tired or full of energy. We experience such mental states but are not aware of them unless they exceed a certain threshold. When that happens, what comes to mind is, *Time for a latté*, or *Time to finally get something done* or maybe *It's time for a little lie-down*. We don't obsess over it. One accepts that states of mind fluctuate during the day and one is content as long as they fluctuate within normal boundaries.

Most of us have a high threshold before we become consciously aware of our state of mind. Taking short-acting drugs lowers the threshold. One becomes aware of slight deviations from an optimal state and obsesses over it. Taking drugs also stretches one's normal boundaries. Ordinarily, to be alert is an optimal state. Amphetamines change one's optimal state to hyper-alert. When it wears off, one feels sub-alert, logy and dull. All this up-and-downing makes one obsess even more.

Elspeth felt that she could control her mental state. If she took the right dose of Adderall, the correct strain of cannabis or an occasional Xanax, she could be cheerful, calm, energetic, focused or blissfully insouciant, and each state of mind was experienced sharply. She developed the bad habit of monitoring her mental state. She didn't regard it as an obsession. To her, it was pharmacologic self-control. Minor fluctuations in her state of mind were to be avoided and were easily manipulated. It suited her controlling disposition.

The problem with stimulants is that they are 'on-off' drugs. That means the patient experiences the positive effects of the drug when it is acting and then the negative effects of the drug wearing off, a few hours later. The danger of giving a stimulant to an OC is that the drug *conditions* her to monitor her internal state; what I call obsessive self-monitoring. Elspeth was OC by nature; the stimulant effect taught her to obsess over her mental state.

> Karl was a successful IT guy. He didn't write code anymore. He was good with people and moved to sales. He did well, not least because of his boundless energy.

> Karl had discovered ADD when he was in college. He got it from friends. Then he went to student health, filled out a questionnaire, and was given a prescription for Adderall. To qualify for academic accommodations, he would have needed a full psychological evaluation, but for Adderall, a questionnaire and a short interview were enough.

> He continued on Adderall after he graduated. Coding was easy with Adderall and Mountain Dew. He could write code for 14 hours straight. Sales were different. Adderall helped him get paperwork done but he found himself using higher doses to keep his energy up and to fortify his spirit. Sales is a taxing occupation, and the software he was selling was getting old. Finally, his primary care doc got nervous with the dose he was using and insisted he get further prescriptions from a psychiatrist. That brought him to our clinic.

Karl was in robust good health and his examination was normal. He spoke well and was an intelligent fellow, but he clearly regarded the consultation as an unnecessary and burdensome exercise. Then we tested him. The results were amazing. He scored well below average on virtually every test. He did worse than my patients with early Alzheimer's. I asked him if he had taken the drug that morning and he said he had. Either he was faking bad or there was something seriously wrong.

I told him we couldn't give him a prescription and that I thought there was something seriously wrong. *You're damned right there is. I'm taking Adderall 30 mg three times a day and this ADD is killing me.* Although I was dealing with an angry man, I had to smile. I've never known anyone to die from ADD.[35]

Karl drank a lot and smoked cannabis to sleep at night. He needed it, I suppose, with all that amphetamine in his head. Like Elspeth, he was obsessed with his state of mind and energy level. Like her, he learned he could control those things by taking amphetamine. Like Elspeth, he was a controlling fellow, and such characters can develop an obsession if the circumstances are right. The ability to manipulate his mental state led Karl to monitor his condition in an obsessive way.

Amphetamines affect mood, cognition and energy. The drug's action is always in the back of one's mind if not in conscious awareness: the mild rush as it comes on, the warm, stable feeling of effectiveness that follows and lasts a few hours, and then the downer that comes when the stimulant effect wears off. Karl was always on or off, and he knew it.

Habitual functional use of amphetamine is a do-it-yourself approach to self-regulation. To some individuals, it is an enticing prospect. The question is, can you do it better than your brain does?

Mental self-regulation is a normal function of neural networks in the prefrontal cortex and a few other parts of brain. It is something that a normal brain does on an unconscious level, responding to external events like a sunny October day, a heavy meal or a crucial interview. Self-regulation is strongly influenced by the signals brain receives from all over the body. The goal is to maintain *homeostasis*, the proper balance among all of one's bodily systems in accord with the body's natural rhythms. One's unconscious brain does that in a gentle way, with slow oscillations between periods of high and low energy, high and low alertness, etc. It sounds nice, but our physiological state is not always accommodating to what we want to do or have to get done. In such instances, an artificial boost is just the thing.

We drink coffee for that very purpose. That's OK, we have decided, because coffee is good for you. It's not a bad functional habit. We are not quite so sanguine about energy drinks, but they are used for the same purpose. Whenever amphetamines have been freely available, they have been used in the same way that some people use coffee, tea or Red Bull.

Later on, we shall spend more time discussing the potential dangers of stimulants when they are used in low doses with medical supervision. The danger apparent in the cases of Karl and Elspeth is the consequence of their effectiveness as stimulants. They turn one's mental state into something to obsess over. The do-it-yourself approach to brain regulation entails oscillations that are not quite so gentle, but with sharp highs that terminate in a withdrawal state a few hours later. Up and down, on and off, high and low; it's an experience that captures one's attention and directs one's subsequent behavior. *Oh, Crikey. My ADD is coming back. I need another Adderall.*

13. FUNCTIONAL USE, DEPENDENCE AND ADDICTION

The difference between Elspeth and Karl was his use of ever-higher doses of the drug. It can turn a bad habit into an addiction. What does that mean?

Karl and Elspeth were physically and psychologically *dependent* on amphetamine. Drug dependence is not a synonym for addiction. Physical dependence means that stopping the drug causes withdrawal symptoms, like the headaches that arise when one stops drinking coffee. Psychological dependence is when stopping the drug, or the thought of stopping it, causes anxiety. Dependence, however, happens with many drugs, including antidepressants and some anti-hypertensives. When regular users of stimulant medications stop the drugs, they experience somnolence and fatigue for a few days, and may feel foggy-headed; they are withdrawal reactions, signs of physiological dependence. But they are mild and short-lived symptoms and less troublesome than withdrawal from caffeine. People who use stimulants intermittently, like ADD kids who only take Ritalin on school days, don't experience withdrawal or rebound symptoms on days when they don't take the drug.

Dependence is not addiction. Addiction is self-destructive drug dependence. It is the compulsive use of a substance in the face of overtly adverse effects. Amphetamine addiction causes adverse effects that are painfully obvious, from meth-mouth to punding.[36]

Elspeth felt compelled to take Adderall and cannabis every day and had withdrawal symptoms if she stopped. But the drugs didn't have overt adverse effects. If she took them for the rest of her life, maybe they would. She was using the two drugs as some people take Zoloft and melatonin. I think Zoloft and melatonin are preferable to amphetamine and cannabis, but I couldn't marshal sufficient argument to induce Elspeth to change.

Was Karl addicted? You could say that he was on the way, if not there already. High doses of stimulants, like his 90 mg of Adderall, disrupt normal sleep patterns, raise one's heart rate and blood pressure, make one irritable and impair judgment and cognitive abilities. He already had some of those problems. He'd have them all if he kept on.

Nevertheless, it's hard to think that Karl is in the same league as a speed freak or coke-head. Regular users of methamphetamine take up to 50-500 mg (100 to 1000 mg of Adderall) as often as *several times a day*. Meth is more potent than amphetamine, it lasts longer and is more toxic. Tolerance to methamphetamine's pleasurable effects develops when it is taken repeatedly. Abusers often need to take higher doses of the drug, take it more frequently, or take it by injection.

But even with methamphetamine, there are grades of using and not every user is addicted. The term *functional use* was coined by researchers who interviewed methamphetamine users. Users gave good reasons for taking the drug: they were more productive, could perform better and functioned normally. Whether they were fooling themselves as well as the investigators is an open question.

It may not always seem so, but the third millennium has dawned upon a world where human beings are healthier and longer-lived than ever before, better fed and looked-after, richer and better educated. Our enlightened species appears determined to turn venerable old beliefs upside-down, perhaps for the better, perhaps not. Having achieved phenomenal success on the evolutionary ladder, our species seems determined to undermine the norms and standards that got us here.

So, our attitudes towards so-called drugs of abuse are changing dramatically. For example, the medical profession has come to acknowledge that we know less about addiction than we once thought. Habitual, functional use of amphetamine is usually not an addiction, although that doesn't necessarily mean it's a good thing.[37]

The Adderall explosion isn't an addiction epidemic, at least not yet. Elspeth and Karl are a new category of amphetamine users. They are habitual functional users, and most use low doses, as Elspeth did, and not high doses, like Karl. They may not have had a medical reason to start stimulants, but taking them every day cultivated dependence on the drug. It doesn't take long for regular users to convince themselves they need the drug. *This ADD is killing me*.

Another category is occasional functional amphetamine users. They don't have a medical reason to take the drug but use it a performance enhancer. They are more alert, less fatigued, and can get more done.

Technically, using low doses of amphetamine intermittently to get an onerous task done, to stay awake when one has to, to fight fatigue and improve performance, is *misuse*, something that physicians decry. Misusing prescription stimulants also means taking them occasionally for a specific purpose: to shed a few pounds, to stay up longer to work or study, to stay alert on a long drive, to get some tedious job done and feel better as you do it. Occasional use may be problematic but usually it's not; that's why people have been doing it since 1929, when amphetamines first became available, and why patients are not unwilling to share a few doses with family or friends.

Is it a bad idea to use stimulants occasionally for such purposes? Physicians may disapprove, but a good number of them used stimulants in just that way during their training. Surveys of medical students and resident physicians in several countries have shown rates of occasional or habitual amphetamine use ranging from 5% to 50% (sic).

Some 'good reasons' for taking a stimulant are not so good.

One will shed a few pounds but amphetamines are not supposed to be good weight-loss drugs. Nevertheless, not a few of our patients believe it is easier to keep their weight down when they are on Adderall. Shedding a few pounds may seem a good reason to a model preparing for a shoot or a bride who wants to fit into her wedding dress.

Few providers countenance taking amphetamine to counter the sedating effects of alcohol and other drugs, staying awake for days on end, or to enhance their mood and have a good time. Recreational users know that amphetamine enhances the effects of cannabis and opioids. (OTOH, terminal patients on high doses of opioids will be more alert and energetic, and will have better pain control, if they also take amphetamine.)

Low doses of amphetamine are safer than high doses, and intermittent dosing is safer than regular use. However, even a single, low dose can precipitate a cardiac arrhythmia or a blood pressure spike. The pressor effects of amphetamine are small and clinically insignificant, unless one happens to be unusually sensitive, and as long as one doesn't have a little aneurysm hiding in his head.

It's misuse to misrepresent one's clinical state to a physician, to fill out the symptom rating scale to induce the gullible fellow to prescribe an amphetamine. But it's also the only way to get a prescription. As we meet the next few characters, you can decide for yourself whether the physician prescribed the stimulant for a good reason or not.

14. OVERLOAD

Functional, non-medical amphetamine use probably accounts for most of the millions of adults who use amphetamines, habitually or not, for supposed ADD. 'Functional' means they have a worthwhile use for the drug. 'Non-medical' means they don't really have a health condition that requires a stimulant. 'Habitual use' means taking the drug every day.

> Marcia was 44 years old, married and with three daughters. She was a nurse with an important job at the University hospital. Her husband was the regional manager for a medical equipment company, responsible for sales and service in seven states. Marcia and her husband were doing well but not well enough to afford a nanny. They had a nice house with a pool, and the kids did well at school. The girls were good athletes, too. The oldest was on a travelling soccer team and would likely get a scholarship.

> The nice house had a crack in the foundation and one day the workmen broke the outlet for Marcia's electric SUV. Her husband was on a trip. She got her neighbor to wait for the electricians because she had a presentation to make to Risk Management and the hospital's self-insurance committee. Her father-in-law was going to take her youngest daughter to ballet but his wife was not well and she had to arrange a back-up. Her laptop was in the electric car and she couldn't open it.

> She took one of her daughter's Adderalls and got through it all. Then she made an appointment.

The word is 'role overload'. Marcia is an executive, mother and wife. She is extremely good in all those roles, including the role of daughter to her senile mother-in-law. Some days, though, she feels she can't keep up with any of one of them; lately, most days. She knows that she ought to find deep satisfaction with every one of her chosen roles. She is a good Christian and knows that she ought to feel joy helping the old lady. Lately, all she feels is frustration and disappointment. Her therapist told her she was stressed out by overload. She didn't have time to continue in therapy so she never found out what to do about it. Then she took an Adderall and knew exactly what she had to do.

'Overload' is part of common discourse, as in role overload, sensory overload, information overload and attention overload, not to mention iron overload, fluid overload, circuit overload and overload policy. It has taken the place formerly occupied by stress, which implies weakness in the one who is stressed. Overload keeps the blame out there. Too many things to do, too much stimulation, TMI. Feeling stressed is a sign of frailty; overload suggests that your superior qualities have attracted a super-abundance of responsibilities.

For that reason, I suppose, overload is a popular topic in business circles, especially information overload. When Reuters surveyed managers in Britain, the US, Hong Kong and Singapore, about half said they wasted time looking for information and another half, presumably the other half, said they couldn't cope with the volume of information they found. They had 'information anxiety', which Reuters concluded was a regular part of most executives' lives. It led to headache, mental anguish and physical illness. No fewer than 61% of the managers said they cancelled social engagements because of information overload.[38]

You experience information overload when you go the store, or to a restaurant, or Starbucks. Psychologists have proven that having too many choices causes "anxiety, cognitive paralysis and impulsive decision-making." You wind up with the lavender oat-milk chai latté when all you wanted was coffee and it cost four dollars more. Information overload is not only a way to evade social engagements. It is a new way to say, *There's a sucker born every minute*.

One should spend more time reading the Harvard Business Review and related screeds, if but for the graphic images: *The data glut we all slog through every day at work simply reduces our attention span and makes us numb to anything that doesn't lurch out and grab us by the throat*. I can imagine Marcia gripped by the throat as she prepares her presentation to the Insurance Committee but it's more likely she swallowed her gum or her goiter was acting up. In fact, if we read further into the topic, we discover that information overload is not a general problem, but that it stresses some people more than others. In other words, some people get stressed out and others don't.

The people who don't are said to be better at 'prioritizing and winnowing'.[38] Of course, that would be a problem for Marcia, who has to decide whom to winnow. She is, after, occupying four roles of inestimable importance. In fact, they aren't roles at all; they are achievements. If she feels she can't give the attention she would like to any one of them, it is a measure of her conscientious nature. We modern humans have cultivated our strengths so effectively we are muscle-bound. There is so much we have committed to do and so much more that we would do if we had a free minute, we can't do hardly anything without worrying that we're not doing something else. Strengths cultivate weakness, and weakness must be pathological. So, Marcia concludes that she must have ADD. BTW, her good husband, Ken, volunteered to take last place on her priority list but said he didn't want to get winnowed.

The lives we 21st century people enjoy aren't a problem. We enjoy health, longevity and a standard of living unparalleled in human history. We have more comfort and leisure in our fabulous homes, and we get more stimulation than is good for us. We may well be overloaded with information and multiple roles but we must like it because we keep doing it. We are happy to be overloaded with things to do, with friends, possessions, creature comforts, and opportunities to overload ourselves a little more.

If Marcia had time for her therapist, she would probably have been told to simplify her life. She could quit her executive position and go back to nursing. But she loved her career. She had been a nurse for fifteen years before she got into management and she took her role seriously. She didn't want her hospital to be run by people who didn't know how to take care of patients. She could hire a nanny but that would take money from the college fund. When her oldest daughter had her third concussion she had second thoughts about the girl playing soccer in college. She could send her mother-in-law to a nursing home but that ran against the grain.

Not many of us, leading lives that so full and rich, will opt for simplifying, to quit the job, move to the mountains and herd goats. We like having 10,000 movies to choose from on any given night and some people even like lavender oat-milk chai lattés. We simply want enough energy to cope with it all.

Marcia felt that she couldn't give proper attention to the important things in her life. By the calculus of ADD science, she had attention overload. That is, her attentional resources were insufficient to the demands made of her. 'Adult-onset ADD' is what they call it. All that means is that she is an adult, never had attention problems before and that now she finds it hard to keep up. Well, the woman needs some help, but it would be nice if her helpers knew what was wrong and why. Marcia told me that she had 'attention overload'. What does that mean?

Attention is an energy-hog. We know that from modern neuroimaging methods that can measure oxygen and glucose consumption in different parts of brain and the activity of enzymes in the mitochondria.[*] During tasks that require

---

[*] Mitochondria are the tiny powerhouses in the neuron that convert energy contained in glucose or lactate to ATP. ATP is an energy-laden molecule that fuels virtually all cellular activities.

focused attention, more oxygen and glucose is consumed and enzyme activity in mitochondria increases. There is no such increase during passive observations while taking a walk, daydreaming or dreaming at night.

Individuals vary in the strength and efficiency of those energetic systems. Individuals with brain diseases such as Alzheimer's are unable to mobilize the resources necessary to focus their attention for very long. Even in normal ageing, mental energy resources decline, and young children have immature systems that can't mobilize sufficient attentional energy. That's why preschoolers have such short attention spans. Most of the attention problems exhibited by elementary schoolchildren are because their energy systems are slow to mature. Mental energy is one more of those things that are regulated by the brain's Central Executive.

As it happens, patients with attention problems, including ADD, have lower levels of energy generation in the relevant parts of brain; also, stimulant drugs increase energy generation. We shall return to this point in later chapters, but I mention it here because it is pertinent to Marcia's problem. She was simply running out of energy to cope with it all. You can call it 'role overload' or 'attention overload'. You can even call it 'adult-onset ADD'. I prefer ordinary speech; call it running out of energy.

In 1943, the Medical Research Council in the UK published A Guide to the Preservation of Life at Sea after Shipwreck. (In 1943, shipwreck was a problem for British sailors.) "Energy tablets (i.e., amphetamine) (1) lessen feelings of fatigue and exhaustion, promote alertness, raise the spirits, and prolong the will to 'hang on' and live; (2) prevent sleep. These effects take about an hour to come on, and they last for several hours, but repeated administration cannot prolong the effects for more than a few days." Benzedrine, the amphetamine people used in those days, was part of every sailor's survival kit.

I knew Marcia because her husband and one of her daughters

came to our clinic for ADD. She told me that she would borrow one of Ken's Adderall's every once in a while, but she thought it would be better if she had her own prescription. She told me that she would probably use one or two pills a month.

I didn't tell Marcia to read the Guide for Survival After Shipwreck. She was a nurse and knew all about amphetamines. I gave her a prescription for Adderall, and it took her a year to use 30 tablets. She only took one when she was at sea.

15. MULTITASKING

One of my patients, Rebecca, said, *Five years ago I thought I was good at multitasking. Now I think I'm taking crazy pills.*

Rebecca was 44 years-old. She was a nurse, too. She had been in military before she went to nursing school and she was still in the Reserves. She needed the extra money and benefits, but she was a Major now, and was responsible for training nurses for deployment. She had a 9-year-old daughter and shared custody with her ex-husband. Their relationship wasn't bad but she worried when the child was with him. He was sweet but not the most responsible guy.

She was also the head nurse at one of the ICU's at our University Hospital. Or, she had been. She left the ICU for a case-review job with a managed care company. It paid more and was less hectic. She said that she used to be good at multitasking but she just couldn't do it anymore. She went to a psychiatrist who thought she was depressed. She came to our clinic because she thought she had ADD.

Rebecca and Marcia were experiencing similar problems at the same stage of life. Their attentional resources were stretched by the many roles they had to play, by all the things that required their attention. For most of their professional lives, the two nurses were able to multitask so efficiently they never realized they were multitasking. Rebecca wondered if she should take a stimulant. *Do stimulants help you multitask?*

Multitasking means doing two things at the same time. Walking and chewing gum at the same time doesn't count; multitasking means that both activities require active attention. Multitasking is working on a report, answering e-mails and phone calls, attending to one's little girl who wants a glass of water and then getting right back to the report. BTW it was due yesterday.

The rule is that one can attend to only one thing at a time, but it's really just a guideline. There is something called divided attention, and psychologists can prove it. A good example is driving your car on a busy freeway and listening to a podcast about adult ADD at the same time. It feels as if you are devoting 20% of your attentional resources to driving and 80% to the fascinating podcast. You are dividing your attention.

In fact, driving is a bit like walking or chewing gum; it is an overlearned skill, almost a habit, and in ordinary circumstances it doesn't occupy much of one's conscious awareness. But when there's a heavy storm or the road conditions are bad, driving occupies all your attention. You would do well to turn off the podcast because you're not listening. Plus, most adult ADD podcasts are garbage.

You can attend to two things at once, as long as one of them is virtually automatic, like folding laundry while your daughter is reading you her essay and asking for corrections. *How do you spell 'chthonic', Mom?* Then you happen to notice that the T-shirt you're folding has a gaping hole. *C-T-H-O-N-I-C.*

What just happened is your habit (folding laundry) suddenly came alive and took over your conscious awareness. Within milliseconds, your attention shifted to the T-shirt. It cost $60. You remember you tore it in the garden last week and wonder why you wore an expensive shirt when you were trimming the rosebushes. You throw it, regretfully, into the rag-drawer. Then, your attention shifts back to your daughter's essay and you misspell chthonic.

Multitasking is easy to do when one of the tasks is virtually automatic. When both tasks require serious attention, the only way to do it is to switch attention from one to the other and then back. Happily, we humans can do it in a fraction of a second. It's because we have (most of us anyway) *cognitive flexibility.* Some people are more flexible than others, cognitively, and the skill tends to fade as one gets older. For a young person, switching attention seems effortless. You've seen kids watch TV and text their friends at the same time. They do it effortlessly. Of course, watching TV and texting are not much more effortful than walking and chewing gum.

Switching attention, however, is an effortful process. It takes a lot of mental energy and can leave you exhausted. Attention is flexible but multitasking is hard work. It also reduces one's productivity; the tasks involved are done less efficiently and mistakes frequently occur. That's why you didn't spell 'chthonic' right. The older you get, the harder it is to multitask. It's enough to make you think you're ADD.

Taking a stimulant, one feels energized and alert. For that reason, it may seem easier to multitask. But like many stimulant effects, it is non-specific. Stimulants do not have a specific effect on multitasking or cognitive flexibility. In fact, they make it harder.[39]

Cognitive flexibility means that it is easier to switch from writing the report to answering a few e-mails and getting your daughter a glass of water without much effort. After the interruptions, you can get right back to the report which, BTW, was due last week. Cognitive flexibility is the essence of multitasking.

The ability to multitask declines with ageing and cognitive ageing, like it or not, begins at around age 35. I shall illustrate by telling you about the Stroop test, a neurocognitive measure of cognitive flexibility, the ability to switch sets easily. The Stroop test is one of the tests on the CNT, a battery of computerized tests we use in the clinic. The Stroop test asks the subject to stop doing what he would ordinarily do when he reads a word, and to do something unusual. First, the subject has to respond to the color the word describes; respond black when the word is 'black'. It's a natural response, and people do it quickly. In the second part of the test, the subject has to respond to the color the word is written in; that is, to say 'red' when he sees the word 'black'. The subject has to switch sets: to suppress the natural response ('black') and activate an unnatural response ('red'). The second part of the test takes more time and the time difference between part one and part two is called the Stroop effect. The higher the Stroop effect, the less efficient the subject is at switching sets. People are most efficient at switching sets, that is, more flexible, cognitively, when they are in their early 30s. By age 40 they are beginning to slow down. The curve below shows the size of the Stroop effect (measured in milliseconds) from our database of 4400 normal, healthy people.

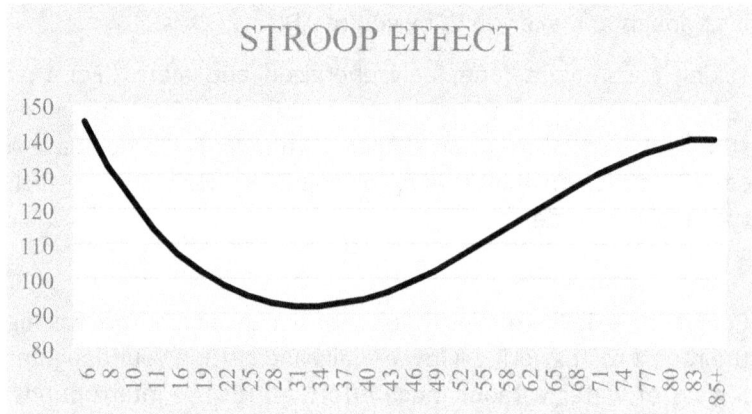

In one's early thirties, the Stroop effect is about 90 milliseconds. At that age, our brains are most efficient and switching sets – multitasking – comes easily. At age 35, the effect starts to get longer and an 80-year-old has as much cognitive flexibility as a child of six. With ageing, it is progressively harder to suppress an automatic instinct – to respond to what a word says – and activate an unnatural one – to respond to the color the word is written in.

Stimulant drugs don't usually improve performance on the Stroop test, and they don't enhance cognitive flexibility or the ability to multitask. For example, our two most recent friends. When we tested Marcia, her scores were all normal, including tests of attention, but she was a bit slow on a test of mental processing speed. After a test dose of Ritalin, her processing speed improved, but her performance on the Stroop test got worse. Rebecca had mild problems with attention at baseline that improved after we gave her a test dose, but she made more mistakes on the Stroop test. In both cases, stimulants diminished the patient's cognitive flexibility. Ritalin made Marcia and Rebecca less efficient at switching from one task to another.

Why, then, did they want a stimulant? They both complained of problems with multitasking, but the drug actually diminished their cognitive flexibility. The stimulant made them feel more alert. They didn't worry about multitasking because the stimulant gave her the energy of a 25-year-old.

Stimulant drugs have specific effects and non-specific effects. Specific stimulant effects can be demonstrated in the lab. Stimulants improve attention, memory and mental processing speed, and those effects can be measured on test batteries like the CNT. The non-specific effects are alertness, increased energy, relief from fatigue and a sense of well-being. When we treat patients with a stimulant, it is for their specific effects on attention, memory and processing speed. In patients, the drugs have a specific effect. People whose stimulant use is functional, like Marcia and Rebecca, usually do it for their non-specific effects.

It's not inappropriate to take a drug that makes you alert and energetic and helps you grind out a report that was due last month but it's not a practice that is medically sanctioned. Unless, of course, you can convince a provider that you're ADD.

Marcia and Rebecca took stimulants with medical supervision. They took low doses and Marcia hardly took them at all. They did well as we followed them in the clinic over the ensuing years. Then menopause happened.

16. BRAIN FOG

Alec was 52 years old and having an awful time with menopause. She had hot flashes and slept badly, and she was getting forgetful. Her mother's mother had Alzheimer's disease and Alec was worried she was getting it, too.

ADD is different in girls and boys. ADD boys are more likely to get in trouble, ADD girls tend to be anxious. Teachers and parents rate ADD boys higher on ADD symptom scales and ADD girls do better at school. As you may expect, boys are more likely to be referred for treatment.

Brain fog, however, is more common in women. Patients with brain fog complain of slow thinking, inability to concentrate and multitask, memory impairment, and 'haziness' in thought processes. Patients with brain fog (aka chemo-brain) may decide they're ADD. Some of them (but not all) get better when they take a psychostimulant.

We don't know why brain fog occurs more frequently in women, although it is a common symptom of menopause and also occurs in medical conditions that occur more frequently in women, like breast cancer chemotherapy, chronic fatigue and fibromyalgia, celiac disease and other auto-immune diseases. *I can't cope with multiple inputs* is the title of an article about brain fog published in the British Medical Journal in 2022. It was about brain fog in patients post-COVID. Persistent symptoms like fatigue and depression often occur in patients who have had COVID infections, even mild infections, and as many as a third have cognitive symptoms. Women are more likely to have COVID-fog.

Because brain fog and all of the medical conditions that cause it occur more frequently in women, the problem has been dismissed as anxiety, depression or hysteria. There is ample evidence now that the condition is not imagined, but a real and debilitating problem. Our tendency to derogate such complaints in the past was based on psychological tests that were too coarse to discover neurocognitive deficits. More sensitive neurocognitive measures like the CNT have demonstrated deficits in mental processing speed, attention and memory, precisely the symptoms of which patients complain. Patients usually don't score in the pathological range on tests, but towards the lower end of normal, well below what they should score based on their education and background. Small differences in test performance, however, can translate into big problems in everyday life, especially in middle-aged women subject to multitasking and role-overload.

We know a lot about brain fog now, except why it happens, how long it will last and how to treat it. It isn't an official diagnosis, but it happens so often in chemotherapy patients, especially breast cancer patients, that the National Cancer Institute has ventured to define it: it is problems with "the ability to think and reason... to concentrate, remember things, process information, learn, speak, and understand". Recommended treatments include exercise, a healthier diet, sleeping better and a host of 'natural' supplements. As I said, we don't know how to treat it.

The subjective experience of cognitive decline is one of the most frequent complaints of women in menopause. Studies report a prevalence rate between 44% and 62% of menopausal women. 'Cerebral fog', as it is sometimes called, affects daily life, with deficits in attention, processing speed, and memory, experiences as lack of focus, slow thinking, and forgetfulness.

Theoretically, brain fog is caused by the abrupt loss of estrogen during the menopausal transition. Ovaries stop producing estrogen one or two years before menopause. About two years after the final menstrual period, estrogen production reaches its nadir. The sudden loss of estrogen has effects on brain. There are estrogen receptors in the brain, and estrogen has multiple effects: it protects against neural injury, enhances synaptic plasticity, hippocampal neurogenesis and long-term potentiation, which is how memories form. Estrogen influences several neurotransmitters, including acetylcholine, serotonin, noradrenalin, and glutamate. Estrogen modulates neural activity during performance of cognitive tasks.

Estrogen loss may precipitate cognitive weakness but performance on cognitive tests does not correlate with estrogen levels and hormone replacement therapy only alleviates the symptoms in some women. Long-term hormone replacement may actually increase a woman's risk of developing a dementing condition.

> The second patient was Louise. She was 56 and had had breast cancer. She didn't have the BRCA2 gene, so she only needed a single mastectomy and then she had a course of chemotherapy. Her prognosis was good, but she wasn't happy. She told me she had brain fog.

'Chemo brain' is yet another term for brain fog. It occurs in about a third of breast cancer survivors and may persist for years. It may be caused by the chemotherapeutic agents themselves, which can affect brain cells. Cancer itself, absent chemotherapy, can also cause brain fog.

Louise knew that brain fog is a frequent accompaniment of cancer chemotherapy and she wasn't worried about Alzheimer's disease. Most cases of chemo-brain, menopausal brain fog and COVID-induced cognitive impairment improve after a few months; the unfortunate few who have persistent cognitive weakness continue to have (comparatively) mild deficits that do not get worse over time, as they would with Alzheimer's. Brain fog patients complain of forgetfulness, poor concentration, difficulty recalling a word or a name (dysnomia), forgetting why you've gone into a room or where you set down your keys or your iPhone. They are benign problems, not associated with incipient dementia. Forgetting what you just were talking about, asking the same question or stating the same thing over and over, failing to remember recent events, and getting lost in familiar neighborhoods are more dangerous signs, and are rarely associated with cerebral fog.

Whether the cause is chemotherapy or menopause, chronic fatigue syndrome or any other condition that makes a person's mind go foggy, the outcome is the same; the problem may just go away or it may persist for years.

A condition characterized by slow mental speed, inattention and poor memory ought to respond well to a stimulant drug. In fact, stimulants are probably prescribed for brain fog patients more than any other drug; at least, they are tried most often. They don't always work. In our two patients, Louisa responded quite nicely; testing showed improvement in mental processing speed and attention, and the positive effects of the drug on her symptoms were felt almost immediately. Alec had no such luck. She didn't like the way she felt when she took Ritalin and her test scores didn't change at all. It wasn't because she was menopausal. We have many other patients who start taking stimulants at menopause and do well. But it is a coin-toss. About half of our brain fog and chemo-brain patients respond to stimulants and half do not.

What does that prove? Nothing, but it does suggest that there are many different things that go wrong in the brain of brain fog patients and not all of them can be corrected by stimulant drugs. It also underscores the unpredictability of stimulant treatment in a number of circumstances when we would expect them to do well.

Finally, the 64-dollar question: why is brain fog more common in women? Frances believes that a woman's mind gets clogged from remembering all the stupid things her husband has done over the years. I think she's just having a joke on her poor, devoted husband. I told her that women and men are different, as if she didn't know. Brain fog occurs most frequently in diseases involving inflammation and immune response, and women have more active inflammatory and immune response systems than men. Obesity and physical inactivity, both more common in women, aggravate inflammatory and immune hyperactivity. I only wish that exercise and a healthier diet could alleviate brain fog, and I haven't met any of supplements that could either.

17. ACTIVE MINDS GROWN UP

I told you there were a lot of people with active minds and I met one today.

> Basil was 48. His wife said he had memory problems. He didn't think so, but he came to check it out. He was tall and fit and he had always been healthy. He was never identified as ADD or earning disabled in school, and he graduated from one of our best universities. He said he didn't like college until the very end, when he finally had a chance to build things. He has been building things ever since, mostly large-scale computer networks. He never had problems at work but his wife said he never remembered anything she told him. He and I agreed that was probably an exaggeration. Husbands have a built-in filter that gets less and less permeable as years pass. It is designed to protect them from idle prattle but will sometimes err and block important information like *Will you call the furnace-man tomorrow?*
>
> Basil's examination was normal and testing showed a very high IQ, which was no surprise. He had a bit of trouble on the Stroop test, taking extra time to get it right, and that was a reflection of his perfectionistic disposition. His attention testing was normal, in the 50th percentile, but it was well below what one would expect on the basis of his intelligence and education. He didn't have ADD, but his attention couldn't keep up with his life.

Children with active minds don't grow out of it. Whether they are diagnosed with ADD or not, or treated with stimulants, they are smart enough to accommodate a world that prefers mediocrity and rewards drudgework. Basil was your typical active mind grown-up. He was high energy fellow, impatient with fools, self-assured and perceptive; but he was easily distracted, especially from what he considered idle prattle. He loved nothing more than to engage the most complicated challenge and devise an elegant solution. He was prone to hyper-focus. If you asked him if he called the furnace-man he would grunt an acknowledgment which might mean *Yes* or maybe *I'll call him tomorrow or at some other time in the indeterminate future* or perhaps *I am in state of hyper-focus and my filter is impenetrable.*

Active minds are perceptive and react sharply to things that we troglodytes don't notice. They aren't heedless of the world, as the absent-minded professor is, but small events will awaken a train of interesting associations. It's distracting.

What happens to an active mind after 40, 50 or 60 years? Good things, usually, but not always. An active mind is an obstacle to chores that are not impelling. We philistines dismiss them as dreamers. They can't be relied upon because they procrastinate. They are perennially distracted by things going on inside their head.

Such individuals are often indifferent students but they are successful when they have the opportunity to be self-propelled. They tend to do less well in corporate environments if they don't have ample room to be themselves.

They are high-energy machines; positive energy is predictive of good health and longevity. But a sensitive, creative mind will be frustrated if it doesn't have opportunities for self-expression. One of my friends, Cliff, was a pediatrician, but he couldn't stand the day-to-day of it. Talking to parents about ear infections for 8 or ten hours made his head feel like an echo-chamber. He left medicine and became an herb gardener. We saw him every week when he delivered fresh greens to my wife's restaurant. He was happy as could be, communing all day with little plants. He was still a pediatrician at heart. I could never imagine him growing big plants.

A wandering mind can grow into a bad habit, especially as the years pass and the high energy that once compensated for it begins to wane.

Active minds are unusually confident; they know what they like. A positive trait, unless what one likes is staying inside his own head. Self-absorption is incompatible with productivity and mutuality. It doesn't make for a solid career or a solid marriage.

Active minds tend to be impatient. Self-absorbed as they can be, they are intolerant of us fools.

Active minds may not have enough energy to take on everything they commit to do. Their adult lives are replete with unfinished projects. It is stimulating to begin a project, to put it together and get it going. Seeing it through to completion is boring. Any MBA can do that. There is always a new project to engage one's energy.

Not every active mind has the opportunity to rusticate as Cliff did. Many are trapped in occupations that pay the rent but limit their creativity. Or with spouses who are impatient with their idiosyncrasies. *James, did you ever think you might be ADD?*

Dorothy could make a pretty good argument to James' doctor and get him a prescription for Adderall. It might get some chores done. He'll be more tolerant of the long, boring meetings at work. He may spend less time playing videogames or reading science fiction.

With Adderall, James quit his job designing data systems for the shipping container company and go into business for himself. His start-up was successful, although he had to up his dose a couple of times. And his investors don't let him run the company anymore.

There are a lot of paths an active mind may take in life, some of them successful in a worldly sense, others in the nest of family or in pursuit of a perfect garden. The path sometimes ventures into ADD World.

So Basil's path crossed mine.   After an interesting discussion that touched on some of points I made in this chapter, I offered to give him a test dose of Adderall.

Interesting, is what he had to say when he came back.   He wasn't surprised that he did better than average on the Continuous Performance Test. *I can see why people like to take the drug*, he said. *You can get things done you hate*. He said he would tell his wife he finally could appreciate what she was talking about. He anticipated she would fly into his arms.

Psychostimulants don't affect long-term changes in ADD patients.   But some few – children and adults – experience a stimulant as a learning experience. *So that's what it's like to have a mind that relishes drudgery*.

Basil thanked me for an interesting day and shook my hand when he left. He didn't want a prescription.

18. MENTAL ENERGY

Marcia, Rebecca and Louisa benefitted from low doses of stimulant drugs by virtue of their non-specific effects. The drugs are energizing and the patients they needed a small increment in mental and physical energy. Most adults who take stimulant drugs likely do so for just that effect.

> Peter was a minister with a new project. He retired from the Church to get it started and now it was taking off. He wrote a self-help book that helped people immeasurably in a way I never could understand. The book was successful and now he was planning an internet-based self-help program. It was a lot of routine work: composing sessions and homework, filming interviews and editing them, making quizzes and then on-line Q&A. His family physician was dubious when he told him he couldn't meet deadlines unless he took an extended-release Ritalin in the morning. He gave Peter a prescription on condition he would see a psychiatrist...

The problem Peter had was growing old and one problem with getting old is energy. The fuel tanks run low. To an old person, well-being is an afternoon nap. Peter was 60, not exactly old, but he wasn't young, either, and he was done with ministering. His new project was stimulating, but he didn't have the energy. With 20 mg of extended-release Ritalin, he did. He was a healthy fellow, more or less fit, and his testing was normal. Nevertheless, he complained that the laborious tasks that accompanied his new project were simply too much and he couldn't sustain his focus. *I can't concentrate for very long, I get tired*, he said. But his problem wasn't attention at all. It was energy.

It's arguable that all the positive effects of stimulant drugs, including their cognitive effects, are attributable to energy.

College students know that. They like stimulants because the drugs let them stay awake and study longer. Amphetamines are like energy drinks; they are 'alerting, revitalizing, awakening and provide mental energy'. This isn't new news. Remember the Guide to the Preservation of Life at Sea after Shipwreck? In the 1930s, when Benzedrine was easily obtained, it was called a 'pep pill' in the US and 'the confidence drug' in Britain.

The most reliable effect that stimulants have on physical performance is to prolong endurance and lessen fatigue. It's because they are energizing. By the same token, the cognitive functions that they improve, like focus and concentration, are particularly effortful. College students take stimulants when they prepare for examinations; they are able to sustain their focus late into the night, free from somnolence and fatigue. If stimulants improve motivation or initiative, it is because they provide a burst of energy. Amphetamines are like ether. If your old car won't start, spray ether into the carburetor. It's a sudden burst of combustion.[*]

Stimulant drugs increase the activity of dopamine and norepinephrine, referred to as *catecholamines*. The two molecules that are activating to brain. Dopamine is associated with reward and movement. Norepinephrine is linked to alertness and attention. Dopamine promotes confidence and well-being; norepinephrine keeps you awake. Both have activating effects in brain and also in soma: they enhance cardiac function and support blood pressure; they both participate in the immune response to infection. In brain, dopamine regulates the initiation of movements and norepinephrine generates wakefulness. They both enhance effortful cognitive processes like attention, memory and the executive functions. There are differences between the

---

[*] Don't do this if you have an electric car. Also, cars built after 1990 don't have carburetors. In fact, you may not even know what a carburetor is. Don't worry about it.

dopamine and norepinephrine systems, but the two are closely related and their functions overlap. When we talk about what dopamine does, norepinephrine usually does it, too, and vice-versa. They are both energizing.

Stimulants are activating and arousing because they stimulate the activity of dopamine and norepinephrine, but those molecules are not the source of energy. They direct neurons (actually, proteins within the neurons) to make energy. Neurons burn oxygen and glucose to generate energy in their thousands of metabolic powerhouses, the mitochondria. It's internal combustion, albeit on a microscopic scale. Mitochondria are small structures within the cell that generate ATP molecules from the combustion of glucose in the presence of oxygen (oxidation). ATP is a molecule that carries the energy that keeps the cell alive and functional; everything a cell does requires energy and brain cells need more than most. The catecholamines let mitochondria know they should inject more fuel into the system.[40]

Activation and arousal require energy, and all the energy a neuron has comes from mitochondria. By increasing catecholamines, stimulants increase natural energy sources. It is the same way the brain increases energy supply in response to strong experiences, such as vigorous exercise, a sudden fright, falling in love or facing an important challenge. Unfortunately, the challenges Peter faced didn't exercise that natural stimulating effect. His natural processes were getting old. He was probably running low on dopamine and norepinephrine; the cells that make those two molecules tend to die off, and mitochondria have a life-span considerably shorter than that of the organism in whom they reside. So, he needed a bit of artificial stimulation.

Most people would prefer to have a bit more energy, and that is why we consume energy drinks, tea and coffee and nicotine, all of which stimulate dopamine. Wiser people eat well, exercise, sleep well and engage in stimulating activities. What's wrong with a small capsule that does the same thing as caffeine and exercise, except more efficiently and reliably and without giving you the jitters or making you sweat? Plus insurance will pay for it.

Too much energy is not good for a cell any more than it is for a person, who will only end the day in a state of exhaustion and regret, having consumed all that energy pursuing injudicious ends. Energy has to be husbanded carefully. To do so, dopamine and norepinephrine stimulate DNA to make CART peptides (peptides are small proteins). CART stands for *Cocaine and Amphetamine Regulated Transcript*. It was originally discovered when animals (i.e., rats or humans) were administered cocaine or amphetamine (thus the name) which, in turn, stimulate dopamine and norepinephrine. CART is a control system with two functions. It facilitates the activity of dopamine and norepinephrine when they are functioning normally but it limits their activity when they become too active. CART peptides respond to stimulants, depending on the dose. When the dose is low, CART peptides augment their effects. If the dose is high, they try to limit them.

The reason we have such discriminating peptides in our brain and other parts of the body is to support the actions of dopamine and norepinephrine when they are behaving in normal fashion but to restrain their effects when their behavior gets out of hand and threatens to be toxic to cells. Too much excitement and too much stress can both stimulate catecholamines in excess. Too much amphetamine generates too much dopamine and norepinephrine, and CART is there to limit the damage that can happen.

Excessive catecholamine activity occurs in some mental disorders, such as psychosis, mania, panic and acute stress. In normal life it occurs in states of fear, anxiety and stress. When such states persist unabated, mental disorders develop. Excessive catecholamine activity occurs when people take high doses of amphetamines; doing so leads to paranoia, psychosis or mania. High doses over a long period of time cause damage to many neurons and death to as many more. The high doses used by addicts bypass natural protective mechanisms such as CART. They produce short-term gains but long-term degeneration. There is a natural limit to the energy enhancement one can get from amphetamine – "repeated administration cannot prolong the effects for more than a few days."

CART is interesting because it demonstrates that our physiology actually likes a certain amount of stimulation. It is there to enhance the stimulating effects of dopamine and norepinephrine. But CART illustrates the limits of stimulation. In the face of high levels of catecholamines, CART is neuroprotective.[41] It protects neurons from their baleful effects. Everything in moderation, they say, and the catecholamines illustrate the wisdom of that old saw. Dopamine and norepinephrine are essential molecules, but their metabolism has to be tightly controlled. When they are metabolized, they generate oxygen free radicals. Cells have a ready supply of enzymes that neutralize oxygen free radicals; CART is another mechanism cells have to protect themselves from oxidative damage. But at high concentrations, and when their metabolism isn't tightly controlled, the toxic by-products of dopamine and norepinephrine damage neurons.

Such events are not uncommon in biology. The best example is molecular oxygen, O_2, which is essential to animal life. In high concentrations, however, O_2 is highly toxic, generating oxygen free radicals that damage DNA and kill cells. It is what is called oxidant stress, and why so many of us take antioxidant supplements.[†] As it happens, dopamine and norepinephrine

---

[†] We probably don't need to, because we animals are protected from oxidant stress by enzymes that neutralize oxygen free radicals. There is no evidence that antioxidant supplements do much good at all, except for the people who sell them. There are antioxidant *vegetables*, for Heaven's sake. What will they think of next?

also generate oxygen free radicals and other toxic residues, and Nature makes sure that they, too, are disarmed before they cause mischief. CART is one of several such protective molecules.

Is there anything wrong with what Peter has been doing? I don't think so. Older people don't have the energy they used to have. Catecholamine systems gradually decline with ageing; dopamine levels decline by 10% every decade past one's thirties, and norepinephrine almost as much. Even one's mitochondria get old. Peter, you can say, is just compensating for ageing-related catecholamine decline. He is also taking a very low dose of Ritalin and he uses it intermittently.

When we tested him, drug-free, his neurocognitive testing was normal. After a test dose of Ritalin, he scored better on tests of mental processing speed. That was re-assuring; at least the medication didn't make him worse, and there was at least a bit of objective data to show that it had a positive effect. It continued to help as we followed him over the next few years. Older people who take a stimulant for energy tend to stay on the drugs as long as they are active. But in low doses, intermittently. Nevertheless, as we shall see, older people are at greater risk for some stimulant side effects.

19. IS AMPHETAMINE GOOD FOR YOUR BRANE?

Stimulants in low doses are safe drugs – *so safe we give them to children*. They alleviate developmental problems that some children have, and they are useful for a number of adult conditions, too. However, stimulant treatment is purely symptomatic. Stimulants are like eyeglasses, providing symptomatic relief as long as the drugs are used. They aren't supposed to have long-term positive effects.

Thus far, we have only talked about symptomatic effects of stimulants. Therapeutic doses cause a transient increase in brain energy and arousal. That improves attention, memory and processing speed in patients with ADD. In normal people, stimulants are alerting and energizing. In both groups, the effects vanish when the drug wears off.

We know that amphetamines are neurotoxic when they are used in high doses. Now, consider a different idea: Is it possible that stimulants have long-term *positive* effects on brain?

I began to wonder about this in 1986, when our research group at UNC published a paper about Ritalin and memory in ADD children. We decided to pursue this novel result in patients with memory disorders. We chose patients who had had traumatic brain injuries (TBI). They are usually young and healthy and, at the time, they were woefully under-served. It wasn't hard to recruit a substantial number of patients and in 1988 we reported that 15 TBI patients improved clinically and cognitively on the same doses of Ritalin we had given to ADD children. Our results have been replicated many times and now stimulants and related drugs are widely used in TBI patients, although not always wisely.[42]

We wondered if Ritalin just provided symptomatic relief to the patients while their brains were still healing, or may it have enhanced the recovery process itself?

In 1988, we thought we were onto something new and original. In fact, scientists had been studying the effects of amphetamine on brain recovery from injury at least since 1946.   However, the studies were done in lab animals, with little consideration of what it might mean for humans who had brain injuries or strokes.

Notably, Dennis Feeney, a psychologist at the University of New Mexico, took lab rats and destroyed their motor cortex – the part of brain that controls movement. As a result, the rats were paralyzed on one side. After they had some time to recover, he put them on a high, narrow beam. Not all of them at once, of course, but one at a time. He never specified what was under the beam but presumably it was something that made the rats hold on tight. Nevertheless, they fell off the beam – the ones who weren't treated, that is. Rats who had been treated with a small dose of Dexedrine were able to make it to the other side. Feeney concluded that the drug helped them to recover strength and coordination in their previously paralyzed side. It helped their brains get better.

Similar experiments have been done by other researchers in rats, cats and monkeys. They were subjected to brain injury or stroke -- the animals, not the researchers. The ones who had been treated with amphetamine or methylphenidate recovered faster.   The results were consistent. Stimulants promoted recovery from brain injury and stroke.

Studies in patients, however were not so consistent.   Most studies have shown that stimulant drugs are beneficial in brain injury patients but studies in stroke patients have been disappointing. Only a small number of stroke patients respond favorably to stimulants. There are several reasons why stroke patients respond less well. They tend to be older, for example, and have additional medical problems that interfere with recovery, while TBI patients, as a rule, are young and healthy, and respond well to stimulants.

We were able to follow the TBI patients we had treated with stimulants and they did well. After a year, we wanted to know if the stimulants were still needed. We discontinued their stimulant medication – we were using Ritalin in these studies. About half of the patients performed poorly after they stopped the stimulant but improved when we gave them a test dose of the same drug. They tended to be patients who had had more severe injuries. They went back on Ritalin and some have been taking it for many years now. The other patients performed as well on a battery of tests as they had when they were on the drug. When we gave them a test dose of Ritalin they didn't improve. They seemed to have recovered at least some of their cognitive powers during the year on Ritalin.

All the patients had come to us years after their injury, well past the time when natural recovery occurs. In the first group, the drugs didn't promote much recovery, but they did alleviate the problems patients had with alertness, attention, memory and mental slowness. They enjoyed symptomatic relief. In the other patients, stimulants seemed to re-awaken the recovery process, just as they do in rats, cats and monkeys. The neurons in the brains of treated animals showed signs of growth and connection to other neurons. Perhaps the same thing happened in brain injury patients.

So, are stimulants good for your brain? If so, how do they do it? Do they only work for patients who have had brain injuries or do they have comparable effects on other patients? Do they have a beneficial effect on brain development in ADD children, and might they protect older adults from ageing-related cognitive decline or dementia?

HOW STIMULANTS MIGHT PROMOTE RECOVERY FROM BRAIN INJURY

When lab animals recover from experimental injuries after treatment with amphetamine, two things happen. One is familiar to us by now: amphetamines stimulate mitochondria to generate more brain energy. Here is something else they do: amphetamines change the structure and behavior of neurons.

We know that stimulant drugs increase brain energy production in certain parts of brain. By stimulating dopamine and norepinephrine, they increase brain metabolism and the production of ATP. It accounts for their activating and energizing effects. It is relevant to brain injury, because following an injury, metabolism is reduced in regions of brain that are remote from the injury.[*] Much of brain goes into sleep mode, presumably because healing the injured areas requires so much energy. The sleeping regions may not remember to wake up.

Dr Feeney showed that amphetamine alleviates metabolic depression. Mitochondria in neurons far from the injury are usually less active than they ought to be. When amphetamine is administered, they become more active. Stimulation by the drug wakes up sleeping regions of brain and allows them to participate actively in brain recovery. As you know, the brain has only a limited capacity for healing an injured spot. Recovery from a serious injury usually happens because other brain regions take over the functions of the injured region. They can't do that if their metabolism is depressed. Amphetamine wakes them up. This effect, however, would only be relevant to people who have had brain injuries or stroke.

There is something else that stimulants do for brain. We know they increase dopamine and norepinephrine at the synapse – the connection point between two neurons. In synapses, dopamine and norepinephrine are acting in the role of *neurotransmitters.* The more important action of the two catecholamines, however, is outside of the synapse. Amphetamines cause catecholamines to be released from neurons, not only into synapses, but also into the *interstitial fluid* -- the watery space between neurons. Dopamine and

---

[*] The word for it is *diaschisis* or *metabolic depression.*

norepinephrine are able to attach to receptors on the walls of the neuron, where they function as *neuromodulators*. Doing so, they incite changes in the internal workings of the neuron.

In experimental animals, stimulants affect DNA in neurons to generate proteins, changing the inner workings of the neuron. Thus stimulated, the neuron sprouts an axon, branches form on it to contact other neurons, and new synapses are formed. When lab animals are subjected to brain injury or stroke, stimulants change the anatomy of nearby neurons, leading them to grow more connections to other neurons. This increases their ability to take over the functions of injured neurons.[†]

In brain-injured animals and possibly also in humans, amphetamines stimulate the growth of the brain's functional elements. As it happens, these are the same elements that are forming during the many years of a child's brain development. They are also the elements that are impaired or delayed in children with ADD.

DEVELOPMENT

Do stimulants facilitate brain development in ADD kids? Probably not. Here is a relevant fact: ADD children treated with stimulants for two years turn out the same as ADD children who weren't treated at all. When they are taken off meds, they are just as ADD as untreated ADD kids. Both groups are less ADD than they had been, because they have matured a bit. Stimulants help ADD children as long as they take them and that's about it. They are symptomatic treatment.

There have been studies to suggest that stimulant treatment corrects abnormal brain structures as ADD children grow up. The results are dubious. Among ADDs, one may find brain abnormalities and they tend to normalize as the children grow

---

[†] Technically, stimulants cause *axonal sprouting, neurite growth* and *synaptogenesis*.

up. However, structural differences disappeared, whether the patients were treated with stimulant or not.[43]

In some ADD patients, symptoms and disabilities persist into adult life. How many, no one can say; in different studies, persistence rates range from 4% to 76%. Whatever the real number is, studies agree on what factors determine persistent ADD. ADD children who grow up to be ADD adults usually have more severe problems to begin with – kids with MBD – or had additional mental problems, like anxiety, mood disorders, OC, or conduct problems. Treatment with stimulants in childhood and adolescence doesn't influence whether ADD persists or not, or whether additional mental problems will occur.

The long-term studies of ADD children are reassuring because they don't show any detrimental effects of treatment. But they do not support the idea that stimulants enhance or accelerate brain development. Stimulants are just useful symptomatic treatments.

Except, probably, brain injury patients and some stroke patients. Yet, it is still possible that amphetamines are good for the brain in special circumstances. Is 'normal' brain ageing one of those?

20. PREVENTING OLD AGE

Low doses of amphetamines activate natural processes to promote recovery from brain injury and stroke. It is true, within limits. It is true in laboratory animals. It has been difficult to demonstrate in human beings who have had TBI or stroke. Still, there may be something to it. Experimental animals are uniform to begin with and their experimental injuries are also uniform. Patients with TBI or stroke are a diverse group and the brain damage they experience is no less diverse. Recovery from TBI or stroke is a complicated process, but the intelligent use of stimulant drugs appears to support it, at least in some patients.

If stimulants help a damaged brain, are they good for the ageing brain? If you're over 50, you've probably experienced the gradual enfeebling of your cognitive powers. You have trouble finding the right word, your memory is not quite so sharp as it used to be and your inquisitive spirit is mostly quenched. It's because the brain accumulates damage as it ages. Normal ageing makes you feel like you are recovering from a minor concussion, except you never do. Normal brain is subject to chronic inflammation, oxidative stress and mini-strokes.[44] The synapses that connect neurons decline in number and so do the mitochondria. Neurons die off, especially the ones that make dopamine and norepinephrine. It all happens with tedious regularity. If stimulants were neuro-protective in adults, they would alleviate such afflictions. They would protect against ageing-related decline or even dementia. Well, do they?

Howard thought so and he had a lot to say about the matter. He took Dexedrine because he wanted to keep his mind sharp and delay the inevitable.

> Howard was 78, retired from his academic job, but he stayed busy, writing books and reviewing papers for learned journals. He still worked as a consultant and, every once in a while, he would give a lecture

someplace. It was usually in Southeast Asia, because his research had to do with a rare condition that is endemic there. I won't give any more details, because he is well-known and you might figure out that 'Howard' is not his real name.* He was also an ardent gardener, a carpenter and he worked on old cars. Several children and grandchildren lived nearby and inflicted themselves with regularity.

I met him when he brought his wife to see me. She was prone to spells and doctors couldn't discover what they were. They told him to take her to a psychiatrist. He and Betsy came to see me. I won Howard's confidence when I diagnosed her spells right off. Someday I may tell you that fascinating story, if I don't forget.

This vignette is not about her, but Howard. He knew we knew a lot about such things, so he decided to share his scheme with me. He said his internist gave him Dexedrine and he took 10 mg three times a week. He admitted that it helped him get through his ponderous correspondence but that's not why he took it. *I think that a small amount of additional stimulation keeps the brain sharp and prevents decline.*

He drank green tea, too, which he thought was a healthier drink than black tea or coffee.† *I drink it all day*, he told me. *But I have a strong cup of coffee in the morning.* He preferred green tea because the catechins and polyphenols therein are *really good for you* but he wanted to make sure he got enough caffeine. He made himself a nice oat-milk latté in the morning.

---

* His real name is Miles.
† Green tea is laden with catechins and other phytochemicals that are real good for you but you have to get used to the taste.

Tea and coffee are stimulating because they contain caffeine, which must be good for you because 80% of the world population drink a caffeinated beverage every day and most of us are still alive and kicking. The four countries with the highest caffeine intake per capita are Finland (329), Denmark (390 mg/d), Norway (400) and Sweden (407) and it's probably no accident that they always score highest on the World Database of Happiness. Apparently, they have trouble staying awake for it. Nevertheless, authorities in the USA and Europe recommend no more than 400 mg per day, about 4 strong cups of the brew, and pregnant women are advised no more than 200 mg per day for fear of low birth weight or miscarried babies.

Caffeine is a stimulant like amphetamine and it increases dopamine and norepinephrine activity, albeit indirectly. Too much caffeine has effects similar to too much amphetamine and excessive doses (e.g., more than 1000 mg) can cause seizures and sudden death, just as a stimulant overdose can. Caffeine has also been studied as a possible ADD treatment. Some studies were positive, others negative, and the drug is hardly ever recommended for that purpose.[‡]

Howard wasn't ADD, for sure, but he knew about the numerous studies that show that coffee and tea have no adverse health effects. More to the point, he cited research that showed that coffee and tea drinkers are healthier and live longer. There is even evidence, he said, that caffeine drinkers are less likely to develop dementia.

There are two reasons why tea and coffee may be good for ageing brain. One is that they stimulate dopamine and norepinephrine, two governing catecholamines that gradually decline in concentration as one gets older. The other is that old people do better if they stay active; so, anything that confers a bit more energy to their otherwise bleak and aimless lives is a

---

[‡] The reason, I think, is that one develops tolerance to the brain-arousing effects of caffeine. Regular coffee drinkers are usually just treating caffeine withdrawal.

good step. Howard's reasoning was this: if I have more energy and if I can keep dopamine and norepinephrine doing what they're supposed to do, I'll be all right.[45] Why, then, did he want to take Dexedrine?

Amphetamine and caffeine have a lot in common but they are not the same. They both are alerting and counter fatigue. They are both energizing, and thus have positive effects on motor and cognitive performance. They both increase the activity of dopamine and norepinephrine, although in different ways. Therein lies the difference. The caffeine effect is indirect and relies on a number of intermediate steps. Amphetamine acts directly on the two catecholamines. That probably accounts for its greater efficiency as a stimulant. It is more stimulating at doses that don't make one jittery or nervous. One is less likely to become tolerant to the positive effects of amphetamine. Amphetamine, simply put, is a stronger and more reliable stimulant than caffeine.

If caffeine is good for health and longevity and if it may delay or even prevent dementia, then perhaps stimulant drugs would have the same effect, or possibly a stronger effect. That was Howard's reasoning and it was not unsound. OTOH, it's not an argument we shall ever be able to prove. The majority of adults who take stimulants are either addicts or individuals with mood or anxiety disorders, ADD or other cognitive problems, or habitual users like Elspeth and Karl. Those characteristics are associated with ill-health and shorter lifespan. Occasional users, like Howard and Peter, are highly intelligent, active and health-conscious; such individuals will be healthier and longer-lived even if they don't drink coffee or tea or take amphetamine 2 or 3 times a week.

I think I've mentioned the neurons that produce dopamine and norepinephrine decline in number as years go by. The remaining cells try to make up the loss but can't quite succeed;

then they themselves submit to the exhaustion that comes from overwork. The result is all the bad things we associate with ageing: motor and cognitive slowing; low energy, low arousal, fatigue and loss of endurance; low mood and irritability; inattention and memory loss. Presumably, these burdens can be alleviated by drugs that increase dopamine and norepinephrine, and especially by stimulants.

In the old days, before antidepressants and the Alzheimer's drugs were developed, amphetamine was routinely used for all these ageing related problems, and also for early dementia. They were as effective as the new drugs are but, as always, a substantial number of patients couldn't tolerate amphetamine. Older people are more likely to have cardiovascular disease, and stimulants can have baneful effects in people who do.

What stimulants provided to those old people was symptomatic relief. No one thought that amphetamine delayed the brain decline that accompanies ageing, and there were no clinical studies, either. But maybe Howard was onto something. He knew about dopamine and norepinephrine, and he knew that amphetamine was the most efficient way to stimulate those molecules. He also knew that low doses of amphetamine promoted the growth of new brain cells in the hippocampus. The hippocampus is the part of brain that registers memory and has the unique property of giving birth to new neurons – about 800 per day in a healthy brain, fewer as one ages and hardly any at all in patients with Alzheimer's disease. All of us could use a few hundred more hippocampal neurons, right?

It's an interesting idea, I told Howard. I agreed with him, that stimulants are probably underused in older people. They are useful for treating late life depression and problems associated with early dementia.[46] Meaningful activities, such as those he pursued, give one a reason to live. And old folk can usually do well with an energy jolt now and then. Stimulants are also mild pain relievers, or at least they divert one's attention from all the aches and pains that come with living 78 years. Be careful on a hot Carolina day, I told him; you'll stay in the garden too long and get heat stroke. A small dose of amphetamine, once or twice a week, might be OK, I said, but there are side effects. Older people are at particular risk for stimulant-induced hypertension, cardiac arrhythmia and heart attack.[47]

21. PERPLEXING CASES

You've probably been reading thus far in hopes of learning something relevant to your life, your children, your no-goodnik brother-in-law or someone else you care about. In case you haven't come across it yet, here are few random characters.

CANNABIS AND ADDERALL

Worldwide, cannabis and amphetamine are the two most widely used drugs of abuse. So, it's inevitable that people will take both – not only addicts (aka substance abusers), but also functional users like Elspeth. Cannabis is legal in many parts of the world and amphetamines are widely prescribed for ADD in many developed countries. What do we know about taking them both?

> Bruce was 24 years old and smoked cannabis every day, not all day, but he probably maintained a stable blood level. He had done pretty well in school, taking Ritalin and then Adderall for ADD. When he was in High School, he started smoking cannabis. When he went off to college he wasn't taking Adderall but was smoking every day. He crashed and burned. He rarely went to class and mostly stayed in his room sleeping or playing videogames. He moved home after one semester and lived with his father, playing videogames and smoking dope. He worked at a supermarket for a while and then he grew up a bit. He stopped using cannabis all day every day and just took a dose at night to relax from the day. He decided to start community college. He was going to go to State and become an engineer. But he knew he would have difficulty concentrating in school...

Bruce's attention problems occurred in the context of social anxiety disorder, a noxious condition that saps one's motivation and initiative. As it happens, cannabis is a favorite drug for young people with social anxiety. In many such patients it has a calming, anxiolytic effect. The reason so many teenagers like to smoke weed is because it's a stage of life replete with social tensions.

Bruce, at age 24, had finally acquired a measure of ambition and wanted to go to college. He was smart enough to make it there, but he did have attention problems and they pre-dated his use of cannabis. You might think that cannabis would only make his attention and memory worse, and it did when he was smoking all the time. Now he was only using it at the end of the day. He had a car and cannabis wasn't good for driving. He knew that when he went to school, he'd have to cut back even more because he had homework to do, but he was reluctant to stop entirely. He had been on a lot of different antidepressants and other drugs, but cannabis was his only reliable anxiolytic. He wouldn't do well in school, though, if he didn't have Adderall again.

> Then, there was Jennifer, a lively and vivacious 35 year old woman who got a GED and worked for Fedex for a while. She took a few classes at a local community college but didn't complete a degree. Now she designed clothes and had a small boutique and styled hair. She split her time between our small town and the West Coast. She came to see us because she had anxiety, especially when she had a lot to do, and that was often. At those times, she had trouble sleeping. She took cannabis to sleep and it was also her favorite party drug. She didn't smoke or drink or use other drugs, even though she ran with a fast crowd.

> Jennifer was smart and creative, but she had never done well in school. When we tested her, her intelligence scores were well above average but she did poorly in tests of attention. We gave her a test dose of Adderall just to test our suspicions, and she did much better on the tests. She also felt calmer.

She thought she might use Adderall when her business got hectic.

My suspicion was that Jennifer had an active mind as well as an active life. Her anxiety only happened when she couldn't quite keep up. She even had a panic attack once. Anxiety treatments never worked for her. But Adderall did. And cannabis.

People like Jennifer and Bruce present a dilemma. They were both regular cannabis users but were healthy and trying to make something of themselves. Like Elspeth, they were using cannabis as other people might use Zoloft or trazodone; they had tried those drugs and thought that cannabis was better.

It's a dilemma that physicians will face more and more often since cannabis is legal in most of the US and all of Canada and freely available in states where it's not. Is there a danger of combining the two drugs, when both seem to have beneficial effects?

Ten years ago, when cannabis users complained of ADD symptoms, our custom was to give them a test dose. If they responded well, we'd tell them to come back in a month. If they were clean, we would give them a prescription. As long as their urine drug screens were clear, they could continue on a stimulant. We continue to be as strict when the cannabis users are adolescents. But today, we see adult cannabis users who use the drug functionally, as people used to use Valium and now use Lexapro, as a man might have a cocktail when he gets home or a dowager, a glass of sherry at night.

We don't know much about interactions between amphetamines and cannabis. They are both broken down by the same liver enzyme systems, which suggests that taking them together might increase blood levels of both.[47] That would increase the efficacy or the side effects of both. The interaction may not be clinically significant or maybe it will kill you. Heart attack is rare in young people but amphetamine users are twice as likely to have one. Cannabis users are only 30% more likely to have an acute myocardial infarction but when they do, it is more serious and harder to treat. People who take both drugs, especially older people, are at higher risk.[48]

Nevertheless, physicians are going to have to get used to what they call California sober – free from alcohol or other drugs of abuse, and stable on a regular diet of cannabis – if only because we see more such patients every day. There are no standards to guide physicians beyond what we used to do ten years ago. Now, we take one patient at a time.

FINDING SOLACE AMONG THE ADDS

The advantage of being labelled ADD has always been, I thought, the ready availability of amphetamines. Apparently, there are additional advantages to membership in the ADD tribe.

> Clara N. was 26, a graduate student at a prestigious University, and had been treated for anxiety since she was 12. She had been in therapy since then and had taken a host of different medications. When she came to see me, she was on an antidepressant, a mood stabilizer, a tranquilizer and Adderall. She thought she was doing finer but she wanted to talk to an ADD expert. She hadn't been an ADD child and her tests scores were all average or above. When I told her that her perceived problems with attention were, in fact, the consequence of anxiety, she broke down. *I finally discovered what was wrong with me! I found comfort in ADD chat groups. Now you're taking that away from me.*

I always thought the most fashionable DSM diagnosis was Asperger's disorder, aka high-level autism. It is a convenient cover for people who are egotistical and socially awkward.* But

---

* The Social Network, Erica: *You're going to go through life thinking that girls don't like you because you're a nerd. And I want you to know, from the bottom of my heart, that that won't be true.*

maybe ADD is in first place.

It used to be that people were discrete about their mental problems. Now, we will hear stuff like this:

> I locked my keys in the car. It's my ADD.
> Sorry, Ma'am, I wasn't listening. I'm ADD.
> I'm so ADD... It must be somewhere...
> I thought I was stupid but now I know it's ADD.

TV has always been good for neurotics and malingerers to bare themselves as victims of this or that and win sympathy and support. On radio, such people come across as whiners. The Internet, however, allows people with ruminative anxiety and self-preoccupation to band together and find solace. They may even fight back.

> Doctor: Ms N., you don't have ADD in the strict sense. You do have attention problems but they occur in the context of an anxious disposition.
> Ms N.: You're kicking my support system out from under me! I'm reporting you to the medical board.

How much easier it is to give her a ten item questionnaire. To every symptom on the list she will respond: *All the time.*

> Doctor: Yes, Ms N, you have ADD. Do you need more Adderall?

The irony is that some anxiety patients do well on a low dose of amphetamine. Before you write the prescription, though, wouldn't you like to know why she needs it?

MANIA

> Leslie was 50 years old, an executive at one the high-powered industrial giants that festoon our neighborhood. She had a graduate degree but had been depressed, on-and-off, since she was a teen-

---

It'll be because you're an asshole.

ager. In spite of that, she had always worked. In her late twenties she had her first manic episode and was hospitalized. Over the next few years, she had episodes of depression and hypomania but they didn't derail her estimable career. When she was 35, she finally stabilized on lithium and a low dose of Seroquel. A few years later her psychiatrist gave her Ritalin because complained of problems concentrating. After the psychiatrist retired, she came to us.

Everybody knows that when a patient with manic-depression (aka bipolar disorder) is given a stimulant, the drug will induce a manic attack. In fact, that doesn't happen very frequently although, when it does, the manic switch can be quite sudden and dramatic. Nevertheless, one can treat a bipolar patient with a stimulant, as long as the patient has been on an effective regime of mood-stabilizing drugs for a long time. And if it's necessary to do so.

In the good old days, before the Adderall explosion, patients with bipolar disorder were among the most frequent patients who came to us complaining they were ADD. Most of them did have cognitive weaknesses when we tested them. In fact, their performance on tests was usually worse than adult patients who really were ADD. So much worse, we thought they were dogging the test to get amphetamine. There was good reason to be suspicious. Bipolar disorder is often under-treated and many patients with mild forms of the disorder aren't in treatment at all. Alcohol and drug use is rife in such patients. They may like the buzz they get from amphetamine. Mania and hypomania convey increased energy, less need for sleep and you can get a lot done. It also conveys a sense of well-being if not euphoria. When bipolar patients are between episodes they may miss the high, but they can experience a bit of it with amphetamine. The risks can be attenuated by drinking a lot or taking Xanax. Obviously, people like that shouldn't be given amphetamine.

We have since learned that cognitive weakness, especially ADD symptoms, are common in manic-depressives. In a study we published a few years ago, more than 40% of such patients were impaired on at least one of our cognitive tests.[49] The bad actors among them shouldn't prejudice a physician against patients like Leslie, who understood what her condition was and took pains to keep herself healthy. She had been stable for many years, and she stayed stable on low doses of Ritalin.

SCHIZOPHRENIA

Virtually every mental disorder is associated with cognitive weakness, especially ADD symptoms. It doesn't mean that every patient with a mental disorder is cognitively disabled but that cognitive impairment is a common accompaniment of every condition.[†]

> Cindy was 18 years old, adopted into a big family, an 11th grader in a special program. She had always been ADD and learning disabled; her IQ was 75. She had been exposed to drugs and alcohol in utero and had breathing problems when she was born. She had been treated with Concerta (a long-acting form of Ritalin) since she was 5. She had problems with anger and aggression, and at age 10 spent a few months at a residential treatment center. When we first saw her, she was taking Concerta, a mood stabilizer along with an antipsychotic drug. She had been hearing voices

---

[†] Every mental disorder, save two, are more likely to occur in individuals with lower-than-average intelligence. The two exceptions are obsessive-compulsive disorder and manic-depression. It's one reason why I continue to use that old term for the few patients with well-defined cycles of mania and depression, in contrast to the vast numbers of bipolar patients, who often just have problems with emotional instability from other causes. *When Earl's meth lab blew up, Crystal, his wife, said,* Them doctors said Earl was bahpolar but he wunt take his Depakote.

since she was young, voices that were usually friendly but sometimes frightened her.

Cindy has been our patient since she was 11. She was able to stay in school, with a lot of help. She was no longer aggressive, but she still heard voices, although they weren't as loud or threatening. We have continued her medications, with a few changes along the way.

What are you thinking, doctor? Don't stimulants cause hallucinations?

They do, of course, if you're inclined to such things, and Cindy was. But even though she continued to hallucinate, Concerta didn't make them worse. When she didn't take it, she could hardly perform at all in school.

Severe mental illness like schizophrenia are associated with profound deficits in executive functioning: low motivation, low energy, poor judgment, short attention span and lack of perseverance. It's only a few such patients who can take a stimulant without getting more psychotic, but there a few. Even among those few, the stimulant may be beneficial for a while, then lose its effect and aggravate the psychotic disorder later.

MAN ON DISABILITY NEEDS ADDERALL TO FOCUS

Leon was injured at work when he was 35 and had two failed back operations. He was followed at a Pain Clinic and took 40 mg of OxyContin twice a day and 15 mg of short-acting oxycodone four times a day. He was also on an antidepressant, Seroquel® to sleep and Adderall. He was sent to me to me to review his treatment. They wondered if he really needed all those drugs. *All I do all day is sit on the couch and watch TV or read my bible*, he said. Did he ever exercise? *I can walk to the mailbox.* I asked him why he needed Adderall. *If I don't take it*, he said, *I can't focus…*

Stimulants are performance-enhancing drugs and if you aren't performing there's no reason to take one. What, precisely, did Leon have to focus on, and what would be the consequence if he didn't? He may have liked Adderall because stimulants tend to enhance the effects of opioids.

If you have terminal cancer and need an opioid for intractable pain, taking amphetamine along with it will (a) enhance the analgetic effects of the pain med and (b) keep you awake and active, if you care to be. Neither opioids nor opioids + amphetamine are good for chronic back pain.

WHEN HE TAKES RITALIN HE CAN GET HIS PAPERWORK DONE

Paul was a surgeon. He had two children who had been diagnosed with ADD and, out of curiosity, he tried one of his son's Adderall tablets. *It was amazing*, he told me. *I could finally concentrate…*

Paul decided that he, too, must be ADD. When we tested him, he did poorly on the continuous performance test, a measure of sustained attention that is without doubt the dullest, most boring cognitive test ever devised. So, he had a problem sustaining attention to a dull, boring task. Duh. He was a *surgeon*.

It's hard to imagine that one could get into an American medical school and complete a competitive residency if one were, in fact, ADD. One can't imagine Martin, Felix or Henry doing it. Almost all the physicians I have seen for ADD had been kids with active minds, like Cam, or were OCs, like Lilly and Milo. Nevertheless, ADD World embraces them all.

Physicians have demanding jobs and have always been prone to high rates of depression, substance abuse and suicide. 'Burnout' is a state of physical, cognitive and emotional fatigue that is strongly associated with depression. It is said to afflict as many as half of helping professionals, including social workers, nurses and physicians. Burnout causes problems with attention, concentration, memory and judgment, just as depression does.

Medicine is a highly sought-after career so the high rate of physician burnout is no less than astonishing. I have a theory why the rates are so high, and perhaps I will share it with you someday.[50] Burnout is usually treated with psychotherapy, but antidepressants or stimulants may be helpful.

I'm not sure whether Paul was burned out or not, but he wasn't depressed. Maybe he had a bad case of overload. He was more than a bit OC but then, just about every physician is OC. He was 55 years old, so maybe he was just running low on mental energy. As it happened, he was already taking extended-release Ritalin. He had convinced his primary care doc to give it to him on a trial basis, on condition that he would consult a psychiatrist. A year and a half later he got around to it.

Paul continued to take a low dose of Ritalin on days when he had paperwork to do. I suppose the drug was alleviating a weakness that he had, but you can't say we were treating a mental disorder.

22. TOXIC EVENTS

I've given you a lot of reasons why you may want to prescribe a psychostimulant. Now, the reasons not to. Amphetamines cause seizures, heart attack, stroke, liver failure, depression, brain damage, psychosis and sudden death.

Notwithstanding, *They are so safe we give them to children*.

In high doses, stimulants, especially methamphetamine and cocaine, are dangerous drugs. We have had ample experience with stimulant overdose and addiction, going back to when Sigmund Freud was a young neurologist. The German army gave soldiers methamphetamine so they would stay awake for the invasion of Russia in World War II. They stopped because of its fearful side effects, including paranoia and violent rage. Methamphetamine was too much, even for Nazis.

Yet, for all the millions of children treated with psychostimulants, such toxic events are virtually unknown. Kids do get a lot of side effects (headache, GI distress, irritability, loss of appetite, tics, insomnia, sedation, anxiety, dysphoria) but they come on quickly and are painfully obvious. In response to such effects, parents stop the drug. The only side effect that parents allow is loss of appetite. The child more than makes up for it when the drug's not in her system.

At one time, there was concern that amphetamines would retard a child's growth. They do, especially in small children who shouldn't take stimulants anyway. It is only a transient effect, though, and the kids catch up. My only warning is not to give stimulants to a child younger than 8 (or less than 30 kg in weight), and especially to avoid Adderall or Dexedrine; small children are much more likely to experience side effects. They get zombified. If a stimulant is absolutely necessary, use Ritalin, a milder stimulant.

In low doses stimulants are remarkable safe. There are no secret, lurking side effects that will spring up months or years in the future. We know this because millions of Americans have been taking them, under pediatric supervision and the watchful eye of social critics, and they have been doing so since the 1960s. Adults have been using the drugs since 1933; no notable health effects have emerged except among high-dose users. The high doses that addicts use are 50-100 times higher than therapeutic doses. Concentrating on the toxicity of outlandish doses only tends to obscure the problems that can arise when people take normal doses.*

Nevertheless, psychostimulants cause seizures, depression, brain damage, psychosis and sudden death. Only in addicts?

LEE HAD SEIZURES

I have known only one child who had a seizure caused by a stimulant. He was 9 years old and moved to North Carolina from California with his mother. He was admitted to my hospital after a grand mal seizure. It was his first; he had never had seizures before. He was taking 80 mg of regular Ritalin three times a day. I never discovered how he happened to be prescribed so much, because his mother had just been hospitalized in another psychiatric hospital. Lee, the child, was treated with an anti-seizure medication for a while, but he never had another seizure. BTW, he didn't need to take a stimulant, either.

The severe side effects of stimulants are associated with high doses. Lee was being given unconscionably high doses of Ritalin by his mother, who had a serious mental illness. He didn't have a seizure disorder or a proclivity to have seizures for some other reason.

----

* The exception is the 'recreational' stimulant, MDMA or Ecstasy, which may be brain-toxic even with a single, low dose.

Package inserts warn that stimulants can cause seizures, and they can, but only at very high doses. In fact, low doses of seizures can improve seizure control. In the old days, when the only anti-epileptic drugs we had were extremely sedating, it was common practice to give patients a small dose of amphetamine to keep them alert. Seizure control usually improved as well.

OLIVER WAS SCHIZOPHRENIC

Oliver had been treated with therapeutic doses of Ritalin and amphetamine for years and then, in mid-adolescence, symptoms of schizophrenia arose.

Amphetamine addicts may develop a schizophreniform psychosis but therapeutic dose of stimulants don't cause schizophrenia. They may precipitate an acute psychotic episode or unmask an underlying psychotic disorder, but they don't cause schizophrenia or manic-depression.

The package inserts list psychosis as a possible stimulant side effect, and it is, but not very often. However, it's not unusual for an emergency room in the vicinity of a college to be visited by a student who took a few amphetamines to study and became acutely paranoid or started to hear voices. A dose or two of Klonopin[†] and a few hours in bed usually solves the problem.

In our clinics, where thousands of patients have been treated with stimulants since 1982, I can only recall a handful of cases of paranoia in children or adults. The symptoms quickly resolved when the drugs were stopped. Patients who have an acute psychotic reaction to amphetamine aren't down-deep-inside schizophrenic, or likely to turn into one.[51]

ZOMBIES

When he took Ritalin he was like a zombie.

[†] Klonopin or clonazepam is a benzodiazepine, the drug class that includes Valium and Xanax.

Stimulants can blunt one's personality. They can blunt a small child's responsiveness, make him too quiet, inert, zombified. Their parents call and say the kid is like a zombie. That, clearly, is not a desirable clinical outcome. It mostly happens in children who are too young or too skinny to take an amphetamine. Young children don't have enough body fat to mitigate the stimulant effect on brain. Because stimulants are fat soluble, in skinny people all the drug winds up in brain which is mostly made of fat. Thus, the patient's brain is getting a higher dose than the prescriber intends. The result is zombification, an intolerable drug side effect. It's another reason to avoid stimulants in children under 30 kg, which, as you know, is 66 pounds.

Adults seldom experience this side effect, not even really thin people.[‡]

IS THIS DRUG LIKELY TO CHANGE HIS PERSONALITY?

Patients sometimes ask if a medication we prescribe will change their personality. I am tempted to say, *Wouldn't that be nice*, but I usually say If *I had a drug that could change your personality I would take it myself*. Such is the hilarity that suffuses my day in the clinic.

Stimulants are occasionally sedating, especially Adderall, and especially in young children. Stimulants can make you sleepy. Isn't that odd? But it happens. At this point during my world-wide lectures on ADD World, I regale the audience with the old joke: *Do your feet smell? Does your nose run? You're built upside-down.*

INDIVIDUAL SUSCEPTIBILITY

My nurse, Debra, wasn't built upside-down, but she had an awful reaction to a low dose of Ritalin. It was about 40 years

---

[‡] Interesting contrast: adults who take SSRIs sometimes complain that the drugs vitiate their ability to experience emotion – *I can't even cry*. Children hardly ever experience that side effect.

ago, and our research team were studying whether measuring the blood levels of Ritalin were related to clinical response or side effects. Most of the research was done in patients, young and older, but in one study we wondered if it mattered whether one took Ritalin on a full or empty stomach. Our research group made the ultimate sacrifice and took a dose of Ritalin just before the six of us gorged on breakfast at the Waffle Shop. On another day, we took it on an empty stomach.[§] We thought it would be a jolly good time but after her first dose, Debra began to cry uncontrollably. She wasn't the kind of person prone to such things.

In our clinics, we administer more than 200 test doses of Ritalin or Adderall in the course of a year. At least once a year, a patient has the same reaction Debra did.

There are some people who just can't abide stimulants, and I have no way of predicting who they might be. Stimulants make some people sad or even depressed. When a student becomes paranoid or starts hearing voices after he takes a dose or two of amphetamine to prepare for exams, it doesn't mean that he has latent schizophrenia. It just means that some people have nasty, idiosyncratic reactions to stimulants.

There are several reasons why some people can't take stimulants. One has to do with the metabolism of the drugs. As a rule, they are metabolized quickly and don't linger in the body very long at all. When we did studies of blood levels of Ritalin, drug levels were close to zero after only 4 hours, which is how long the effects of regular (i.e., not extended release) Ritalin usually last. But we also found that blood levels of Ritalin were quite variable; the same dose would generate high blood levels in some people and low levels in others. Presumably, people with higher blood levels would be more prone to side effects.

[§] It doesn't matter if you take Ritalin on a full or empty stomach. In either case, blood levels are the same. Most kids, especially little ones, should take a stimulant on a full stomach. Otherwise they may get a stomach-ache.

It doesn't stop there. Stimulants work because they stimulate the activity of dopamine and norepinephrine. Those two small molecules punch well above their weight when it comes to affecting brain function. For that reason, their activity is under exquisite control, involving messenger RNA, a number of enzymes and feedback mechanisms.[52] Remember CART?**

Biological activity at this level of complexity guarantees that individuals will differ in how they respond to drugs like amphetamine. There was something about Debra's biology that made her cry when she took Ritalin. Most times, her biological activity was cheerful and agreeable.

For the same reason, stimulant drugs have unpredictable effects on depression. When antidepressants don't completely alleviate a patient's depressive symptoms, stimulants may augment their effects and allow a patient to achieve remission. Or they may increase a depressed patient's unhealthy ruminations and lead her to focus on the negative. Certain forms of depression that are characterized by apathy, especially in old people, may respond nicely to a low dose of stimulant. Stimulants are not good for depressed patients who may be suicidal.[53]

** What does CART stand for?
  1. Catecholamine Activity Regulatory Transcriptase.
  2. Cleveland Area Rapid Transit.
  3. Cocaine- and Amphetamine-Regulated Transcript.
  4. Can't Always Remember Things. I'm so ADD!

23. SUDDEN DEATH

Sudden death is an undesirable drug side effect although, I suppose, preferable to a painful lingering death. Never having experienced either, at least not yet, I can't hold myself to be an expert. I was, however, elected in my High School Yearbook to be *Likeliest to be found dead, nude, in a cheap motel*.

Be that as it may, I can say with assurance that it is vanishingly unlikely that your child will die because he or she is taking a stimulant. If *you're* taking a stimulant... well, I can't be sure.

The Adderall package insert carries this warning:

MISUSE OF AMPHETAMINE MAY CAUSE SUDDEN DEATH AND SERIOUS
CARDIOVASCULAR ADVERSE EVENTS

Sudden death has been reported in association with CNS stimulant treatment at usual doses in children and adolescents with structural cardiac abnormalities or other serious heart problems. Although some structural heart problems alone may carry an increased risk of sudden death, stimulant products generally should not be used in children or adolescents with known structural cardiac abnormalities, cardiomyopathy, serious heart rhythm abnormalities, or other serious cardiac problems that may place them at increased vulnerability to the sympathomimetic effects of a stimulant drug.

Sudden deaths, stroke, and myocardial infarction have been reported in adults taking stimulant drugs at usual doses for ADHD. Although the role of stimulants in these adult cases is also unknown, adults have a greater likelihood than children of having serious structural cardiac abnormalities, cardiomyopathy, serious heart rhythm abnormalities, coronary artery disease, or other serious cardiac problems. Adults with such abnormalities should also generally not be treated with stimulant drugs.

Similar warnings are found in all the stimulant drug package inserts. Here is the back-story:

In 2006, FDA medical officers reported they had received, over a few years, reports of 25 sudden deaths in people taking stimulants. The deaths were mostly children. When they analyzed millions of health records, it appeared that stimulants increased the risk of strokes and cardiac arrhythmias in children and adults. At the time, about 4 million Americans were taking a stimulant, mostly for ADD.[54]

The reactions were sharp. A cardiologist at the Cleveland Clinic expressed "grave concerns about the use of these drugs and grave concerns about the harm they may cause" and an article in the Journal of American College of Cardiology suggested that "ADHD medications should be prescribed only after safer options, such as regular exercise and omega-3, have been considered and/or tried." (One good reason not to ask a cardiologist to treat your kid's ADD.)

The American Heart Association recommended an electrocardiogram (EKG) before any patient was given a stimulant. The American Academy of Pediatrics demurred, arguing that sudden cardiac death in persons taking medications for ADD is a very rare event and occurred at rates no higher than in the general population of children and adolescents. There was no reason to believe that routine EKG screening before beginning medication for ADHD treatment would prevent sudden death.[55]

Sudden cardiac death is an undesirable drug side effect but it also a fact of life; it happens in old people, adults, adolescents, children and babies. In children, treatment with a stimulant is associated with 1 or 2 sudden cardiac deaths per million person-years. By comparison, this is the annual incidence of sudden death in US children:

Age 0-2	21 per million person-years
Age 3-13	6.1 per million
Age 14-24	14.4 per million
Age 25-35	44.0 per million[*]
Stimulant Treatment	1-2 per million

Sudden death in children and adolescents is rare. Most young people with sudden cardiac death have underlying heart disease, most commonly hypertrophic cardiomyopathy and coronary artery anomalies. About 25% of cases occur during sports – 23 per million per year. The higher risk of sudden death in athletes was strongly correlated with underlying cardiovascular disease.

What about stimulants + sport? Studies of sudden cardiac death in athletes establish risks from anabolic steroids, ephedrine and cocaine, but not amphetamines. There is a theoretical risk that the amphetamine effect on norepinephrine might increase the likelihood of arrhythmia in an over-exerted heart. But more than 12 million Americans play an organized sport, and there must be at least a million ADDs among them. Sudden cardiac deaths in young athletes almost always attract attention. If there were an association with stimulant drugs, I think we would know by now.

One of the two cardio-pulmonary arrests that have occurred in our patients occurred in a young woman who was taking Prozac and higher-than-prescribed doses of Dexedrine during practice for her college swim team. The second was a sixteen-year-old who continued to take Adderall when she had acute influenza. Both events occurred at a time when our clinics were doing routine EKGs before we prescribed a stimulant. Did the stimulant play a role in those events? I don't know. Both young women, thankfully, survived without consequences. No underlying cardiac pathology was discovered.

---

[*] You will find different rates in different publications, but they are all well above 1 or 2 per million.

The American College of Cardiology "rejected the notion that the administration of potent sympathomimetic agents (i.e., amphetamines) to millions of Americans is appropriate." That was in 2006 and nobody seems to have been listening. We routinely referred children to pediatric cardiologists when there was an EKG abnormality that troubled us. I can't remember one who advised us not to prescribe a stimulant.

I can't be as sanguine about cardiovascular risk in adults. Adults are different. They may be less inclined to strenuous sports but they are, as a group, less healthy than young people.

Kids take low doses for a few years. They are more likely to take Ritalin, mostly on school days. Adults tend to take higher doses of Adderall, Vyvanse or one of the other amphetamines, every day, for years on end.

Adults are more likely to take additional drugs. They are also likelier to have cardiovascular risk factors, to smoke, drink too much and abuse drugs.

Stimulants raise heart rate and blood pressure, a bit more in adults compared to children. It's usually only a small increase, and of no clinical importance in kids. In adults, over a lifetime, even a small BP increase carries a toll.

Some adults experience higher blood pressure increases even after a single dose of a stimulant. Others will experience palpitations, arrhythmias, tachycardia or EKG abnormalities. Such events rarely occur in children.

Atrial fibrillation is a particularly nasty cardiac arrhythmia, and one that is increasing in the population, probably because we're all getting older. The lifetime risk of Afib is 20-40%. Amphetamine can precipitate or aggravate the arrhythmia.[56] A history of Afib is an absolute contraindication to stimulant treatment.

In the fifty years since 1960 cardiovascular death from heart attack or stroke declined dramatically in the USA and other developed countries. The beneficial trend reversed after 2007. The increase is usually attributed to obesity, increased blood pressure and diabetes. However, during that time span, *stimulant prescriptions for adults have increased fivefold*.

Stimulants may be safe when we give them to children, but they are not innocuous in adults. Credible reports document increased risk for transient ischemic attack and sudden cardiac death in adults taking prescription stimulants. Patients over 65 are prone to heart attack, especially in the first few months after they start taking a stimulant.

We know it's not a big risk to prescribe amphetamine to adults, especially if the patient has no signs of cardiovascular disease and no cardiac risk factors. Whether the risk is small or medium depends on the patient and whether he's lucky.[57]

Eleven million American adults are participating in an interesting natural experiment. The research question isn't whether amphetamines are as safe in adults as they are in children. We know that they are not. The question is, How many casualties will there be?

24. PERSONAL USE

In 2007, the journal <u>Nature</u> conducted an online poll of readers and asked if they would consider "boosting their brain power" with drugs. 1,400 readers from 60 countries responded to the online poll. It was an interesting exercise, not a scientific study. People who read <u>Nature</u> tend to have advanced degrees in science and aren't representative of the general population.

Among those well-educated and presumably respectable readers, one in five said they had used drugs for non-medical reasons to stimulate focus, concentration or memory. Most of them took Ritalin, Adderall, Dexedrine or modafinil, but there were some real chestnuts like centrophenoxine, piracetam and ginkgo biloba. No fewer than 80% of the respondents wrote that healthy adults should be able to take the drugs if they wanted to but 86% thought that children under 16 should be restricted. However, one-third said they would feel pressure to give cognition-enhancing drugs to their children if other children at school were taking them. In essence, they were endorsing purposeful or functional drug use. From here on we shall call it *personal use*.

In 2008, <u>Nature</u> published a commentary in response to the survey, by seven distinguished scientists. They wrote that "We should welcome new methods of improving our brain function... Mentally competent adults should be able to engage in cognitive enhancement using drugs." With what could only have been tongue-in-cheek, they raised a call for "legislative action to channel cognitive-enhancement technologies into useful paths."[58]

I am not aware of legislators heeding the call, but fifteen years thence, amphetamines are freely available: from friends and relatives but mostly from providers who diagnose ADD to anyone who looks halfway normal and complains he can't focus.

The extraordinary increase in amphetamine prescription is reflected on high school and college campuses. College students have little difficulty getting a stimulant prescription at Campus Health. All they have to do is tell a good story, preferably in tears. *I'm going to flunk out. I can't focus on my work. I've always been able to compensate for my ADD, but now I've hit a wall.* Why they bother with the charade, I don't know. They can get stimulants easily enough from friends or family. Estimates are that 5-10% of high school students and 5-35% of college students use stimulants obtained without a prescription. Among college students with stimulant prescriptions, 25-60% shared their medication. Medical students with prescriptions must be equally generous. As many as 50% of medical students in some schools have used amphetamines obtained without a prescription.[59]

University students are the best-studied group of personal users. Only a small percentage use stimulants to get high. Most of them take stimulants purposefully: to concentrate harder, to stay alert and to study longer without getting tired. They also drink coffee and consume energy drinks, which are not nearly so energizing as amphetamine.

Nature readers are smart people, and they know that prescription stimulants are readily available. They must also know how to get all the Ritalin, Adderall, Dexedrine, modafinil, centrophenoxine, piracetam and Gingko biloba they need. They are also taking an honest position. Why should I have to pretend to be ADD? It is a reasonable personal decision to take amphetamine in low doses to enhance my cognitive powers. The drugs are so safe, after all, *we give them to children*.

It's reasonable, but is it right?

It's *unfair*, you might say. It gives drug users an unfair advantage over people who prefer to respect the law and medical convention. That's why stimulants are banned in athletics. They increase physical speed as well as mental speed and physical energy as much as mental energy and they give users an unfair advantage.

Technically, personal use is *drug abuse*, even if it is comparatively safe. Marcia, Rebecca and Peter would be breaking the law if they used their children's Adderall or Ritalin. Instead, they got it from a clinic. Yet prescribing a stimulant for the problems they had is not in accord with FDA indications. Technically, their physician was abusing his prescribing privileges.

It's not *natural* to take a drug to enhance one's powers. Not only is it cheating, it is unnatural and leads to abuse of other drugs and ultimately to addiction.

It is *dangerous* to use stimulants without medical supervision.

The counter to these arguments is that they aren't convincing. At least not to the millions who consume stimulants or to providers who prescribe them on the flimsiest of pretexts. The personal use of stimulants is widespread and growing fast. It is largely countenanced by many physicians.

The best argument against personal use is what happens to the population when mind-altering substances are freely available. Releasing vast quantities of amphetamines into the population at large only increases the numbers of people who take the drugs in harmful ways, or who are harmed by the drug even if they take it judiciously.

There is another reason <u>Nature</u>'s position isn't right. It is wrong.

The eminent scientists who advocate stimulant drugs to enhance their mental powers need to be better informed. They wrote that "these drugs increase executive functions in patients and most healthy normal people, improving their abilities to focus their attention, manipulate information in working memory and flexibly control their responses... A modest degree of memory enhancement is possible with the ADHD medications." It is a compelling argument. If only it were true.

PART THREE

WHAT DO AMPHETAMINES DO?

Psychostimulants *are* smart drugs. They are the only molecules that reliably improve attention, memory and psychomotor speed. In patients, they are quite effective over the long-term. In normal, healthy people, they have small, short-term effects. They exercise their beneficial effects by generating mental energy and enhancing the efficiency of neuronal communication. They affect the regulatory apparatus of the brain, the central executive. The effects are amply demonstrated in studies of normal, healthy volunteers. However, the positive cognitive effects of psychostimulant drugs in normal people are not at all impressive in the real world, and they are small even in laboratory studies.

If the cognitive effects of amphetamines in normal people are so small, why do so many normal people like to take them?

25. WHAT STIMULANTS DO (ATTENTION)

Brandon was an entrepreneurial High School student who looked after the pharmaceutical needs of his schoolmates, at least with respect to stimulant drugs. He didn't sell cannabis, except to his friends. *I don't want to get in trouble*, he said. I won't go into all his sources of supply, but he had his own prescription from a psychiatrist and he also got stimulants from several internet Telepsychiatry companies. He sold Adderall by the pill at a substantial markup. When he was caught, he was sent to me for a court-ordered examination.

There was nothing wrong with Brandon beyond a bad case of bad judgment, risk-taking and disrespect for the law. He was an agreeable young man who expressed the obligate measure of contrition although I didn't trust he wouldn't get back into the pill trade as soon as he thought he could get away with it. As he saw it, he was doing well by doing good.

I asked him why it was a good idea to sell Adderall to other kids. I expected him to say, *You don't expect me to give it to them, do you?* He was relaxed with me by then, relieved that I probably wasn't going to recommend a long prison term, and he was clearly full of himself. He said, *It helps them.* He said that his customers do better on tests because they can study longer and remember better. They can pay attention in class, especially if they have been partying the night before. They feel better when they take the drug. He acknowledged that some kids bought Adderalls so they could drink more without passing out, but only a few of his customers did that, and if he found out he made them promise not to do it again. And, he said, the drug was safe. *It must be safe. My pediatrician gave my brother Adderall when he was seven years old. If it's safe to give to a little kid to take every day, what's wrong with taking one or two when you have to get something done you hate.*

Brandon had a thoroughly modern view of ADD. He told me, *ADHD. Everybody in my school has it.*

What Brandon lacked in obedience to medical and legal norms, he more than made up for by his quick wit and powers of observation. He knew what amphetamines do. *They help kids pay attention*. Then I asked him, just for fun, what attention was. He said, *Everybody knows what attention is*. Everybody does, of course, because we do it all the time. Even when we're distracted, we are attending to something.[60]

Well, maybe we don't do it *all the time*. Daydreaming, our minds wander without lingering very long on anything. Dreaming at night is like participating in a movie that runs along on its own script. They are the rare times when conscious awareness is not governed by attention. In both cases, we are aware but only in a vague and passive way. Attention, however, is not vague. It has clarity, as if one's mind were a spotlight shining on one particular thing. Attention is not passive either. It is an active process that always requires mental energy. Attention is always effortful.

Attention has a lot of work to do. It is the way brain controls what enters conscious awareness.   Awake or asleep, brain is bombarded with data from all our senses and from the afferent nerves that monitor what's going on within the body. Information overload, indeed.   Brain has to be good at 'prioritizing and winnowing'.

Attention is a filter that winnows almost all that information, ignoring it entirely or consigning it to automatic processing. Attention filters irrelevant and unimportant things. In essence, attention chooses one thing out of the millions of sensations that enter one's brain.

Attention prioritizes by attending to just one thing at time. Attention is limited like a spotlight that can illuminate only one thing at a time. It seems old-fashioned, just doing one thing at a time, but it's the only way we can get anything done. And if something comes up, attention is flexible. We can switch attention in an instant from one thing to another.

All this is *work*. It is effortful and consumes mental energy. Stimulants improve attention because they generate a bit more mental energy to help one do the work. The attentional spotlight is brighter and the filter is more efficient. Stimulants make it easier to pay attention to one thing. At higher doses, they force you to pay attention to just one thing.

The conventional explanation of stimulant effects is that they increase dopamine and norepinephrine activity, especially in the prefrontal cortex. It's true, they do, but why does that improve attention? Because they increase energy generation within brain cells and they increase the efficiency with which energy is conveyed within neural networks. In other words, they are energy drugs.

Stimulants don't improve every aspect of attention. Attention has many forms and aspects. There is 'top-down' attention, when we choose to concentrate on a particular thing, or we're forced to. There is also 'bottom-up' attention, when your attention is directed by some external event, like a crash in the next room, a bird singing outside the classroom window or a teacher yelling, *Thomas, pay attention!* Stimulants improve top-down attention but they don't improve bottom-up attention; they may actually make it worse.

Examples of top-down attention are selective attention, which is focus. Scanning attention is search. Sustained attention is concentration or vigilance. Sustained attention is the most effortful of all, and stimulants are best at improving it. They are so good that high doses can induce a state of 'hyperfocus' when one is so ensconced in something, it is hard to switch attention to something else. Hyperfocusing means one is cognitively *in*flexible. In fact, stimulants don't help cognitive flexibility or switching attention. They do the opposite. They cause 'hyperfocus'. One is less distractible, but also less receptive to bottom-up attention.

Consider this homely example: you are ensconced in a videogame. Then your spouse says, *What time do you want dinner?* You don't answer; her words haven't registered in your cognitive awareness. You hardly realize she is there. The consequence of such breaches in conjugal intercourse is predictable. You are compelled to make an abject apology and abandon your game at the most crucial moment. Further atonement is necessary after you are told you were called several times and that dinner is cold. Having read these pages, you would have warned your mate that videogames are so immersive they capture your attention and put you into a state of hyperfocus. It won't help, of course, if she thinks you spend too much time playing videogames.

Stimulants capture your attention as a good videogame does. They also make it harder to shift attention to something else. Stimulants make you less distractible. The price to pay is hyperfocus.

Attention is not an autonomous function. It relies on a steady supply of mental energy. It functions best when we are in an optimal mental and physical state, well-rested and at an optimal level of arousal. It's hard to concentrate when one is sleep-deprived or fatigued or sick or preoccupied. One of the earliest signs of Alzheimer's disease is the inability to concentrate very long. It's because the dementing brain is in a state of energy failure. Even in normal ageing, mental energy resources decline and so does the ability to concentrate. Young children have immature systems that can't mobilize sufficient attentional energy. That's one reason why young children have short attention spans.

Stimulants improve attention by increasing the supply of mental energy in the prefrontal cortex, the brain's central executive. They improve alertness, motivation, mental speed, motor coordination and endurance by the same mechanism. They increase the activity of dopamine and norepinephrine in the brain regions that regulate all those functions. Dopamine and norepinephrine stimulate brain cells to function more energetically. All that mental energy floating around in your head makes you feel good; that is why stimulants enhance your sense of well-being.

Stimulant drugs improve attention, especially focus and concentration, in patients with ADD and with cognitive weaknesses from brain injury, incipient dementia and 'brain fog'. In normal, healthy people they have the same effect. In patients, the stimulant effect is sustained. In non-patients, it isn't. They become tolerant to the cognitive benefits of a stimulant.

It's not a good idea to extrapolate from the beneficial effects of stimulants in patients to their functional use in normal, healthy people. In patients, stimulants correct a deficiency. ADD patients are chronically under-aroused, a condition that can be measured with an electroencephalogram. Brain arousal is a measure of mental energy. Treating ADD children with a stimulant improves brain arousal and normalizes their EEG.

In normal, healthy people no such deficiency exists. In the short-term, they enjoy amphetamine effects on attention, memory and processing speed, alertness and motivation but the effects are not carried over into the long term. One develops tolerance.

Tolerance to stimulant effects in normal, healthy people is well-known. The best example is weight loss. In adults, stimulants reduce appetite and cause weight loss. After a week or two, appetite returns to normal and weight returns to baseline. The only people who use stimulants to lose weight now are models who have to shed five pounds for a big shoot next week.

Stimulants reduce the need for sleep. Then, after 2 or 3 days, there is an enormous sleep-debt to pay back.

Stimulants make you feel energized and promote a sense of well-being, or even euphoria. I wish it were true. The effects last for a week or two. The only way to sustain the effects is to take ever-increasing doses. That is what amphetamine addicts do. Ultimately, they crash or go crazy and kill somebody.

A 'mentally competent adult' is advised to take Adderall because it is a 'cognitive enhancer'. It improves one's ability to concentrate. Well, if it were true, I would take it myself. In fact, within weeks, a healthy brain has enjoyed about all the cognitive enhancement it can stand. It adjusts to the external source of stimulation (remember CART?). The healthy brain has many such mechanisms that bring it back to its usual baseline. With a steady supply of an external stimulant, it simply tunes down its natural sources of arousal and mental energy.

With habitual use, brain adjusts to a steady supply of external stimulation and turns down the natural systems that usually do that job. If you take an occasional dose of amphetamine, as Marcia does, what happens is *external stimulation + normal brain*. The drug has a net positive effect.

ES + NB > MORE ENERGY, MORE ALERT

If you take amphetamine habitually, as Elspeth did, what happens is *external stimulation + normal brain, tuned down*. Net effect, zero.

ES + NBTD > YOUR OFF-DRUG BASELINE

When normal, healthy individuals use the drugs habitually, they feel they need to take them. It is because they are treating the downer that comes from stimulant withdrawal. It takes a couple of weeks for their normal brain to tune itself back up.

26. MENTAL SPEED

Runella was 24 years old and graduated two years ago. She was working in the library and trying to get into law school. *My grades are OK*, she said, *But I don't do well on standardized tests. I got extra time when I took the SATs, but the LSATs are different. They say I need a medical diagnosis.* I said I had never met a Runella before. She told me it was her grandmother's name. She was a healthy young woman and she spoke well but in a soft voice and slowly. Her examination was perfectly normal and testing indicated above-average IQ and normal attention. Her reaction times, however, were well below average and she did poorly on tests that required speed. She also had mild problems when I examined her fine motor coordination.

Runella had a learning disability that is not widely recognized. Her mental processing speed was slow. She was born with the trait of mental slowness and it remained with her. She was not unintelligent; she got good grades in college. She didn't have any of the common learning disabilities, like reading (dyslexia), math (dyscalculia) or writing (dysgraphia). She wasn't ADD. It was her thinking that was slow and it showed up on a number of our tests. Because she was a smart girl, she didn't need special help in school; she would plod along and study for long hours. She did poorly on standardized tests like the SAT because they are *timed* – everyone gets just so much time to answer the questions.

She had made it on her own for a long time but now she needed help. She was stymied in her applications to law school. I wrote a letter recommending extra time on the LSAT, asking if they would concede 30 more minutes. I wasn't optimistic. The legal profession, in my experience, has been the least accommodating to disabled students, in the LSAT, law school and especially the Bar examination.* Also, the authorities who preside over the world of learning disabilities don't recognize a disability in mental processing speed.

Then I told her I had something that might help; I gave her a test dose of Ritalin, and her speed improved substantially, although only to the lower limits of normal.

Mental processing speed is how fast the brain can think, how fast brain is able to acquire information, analyze and act on it.[61] To put it in perspective, simple reaction time -- *Press the button as soon as you see the light go on* – is around a fourth of a second, or 250 milliseconds. Reaction to a painful event like pulling your hand away from a hot griddle is considerably faster, 20-30 milliseconds. You react to the hot griddle well before you are aware of what happened because conscious awareness is not involved in the reaction. You pull your hand away, say *Oh drat* and only later say *I burned my hand*. We humans would be in a sorry state if the sequence were reversed: *I am burning my hand*, then *Oh drat*, and only then pulling your hand back. Reacting to a painful stimulus, or the threat of one, is virtually automatic. We do it as fast as little animals do because we bypass conscious awareness.

The Necker cube below will give you an idea how long conscious awareness needs to do something a bit more complicated than pressing a button when the light goes on.

---

* That's just my experience, and maybe North Carolina is an outlier. I would tell you that my state has fewer lawyers per capita than any other, but there are already too many people moving here.

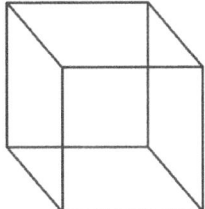

You've seen this one before, and it can be perceived in two different ways. Perception is conscious awareness, and most people need 2 seconds to reverse the image. Two seconds versus 20 milliseconds -- conscious awareness is not very fast.

The speed of mental processing is faster in some people than in others. We are not sure why, but it probably has to do with the way brains are wired. Individuals differ in the anatomy of their neurons and the efficiency with which they connect to form effective neural networks. Something about how Runella's brain was wired endowed her with high intelligence, strong motivation and resilience. For a reason we don't understand, her central processing unit ran slowly. We were able to alleviate the problem but not correct it. We used a drug that enhanced the activity of a molecule in her brain, dopamine, which has a reliable effect on mental processing speed.

Like other neuromodulators, dopamine floats in the watery fluid that surrounds nerve cells. Floating about, it finds receptors in the axons and dendrites of neurons – receptors that are not in the synapse. Once dopamine binds to one of those receptors, it sets in motion a number of changes within the neuron itself. It affects the way proteins and ions behave and expresses activity in the neuron's DNA. It changes the internal workings of the neuron. Once those changes are made within the neuron, neuronal speed and accuracy increases.

Although they usually don't act in synapses, neuromodulators like dopamine influence the strength of chemical neurotransmission in the synapse. They make it easier for neurons to synchronize their firing. They improve the signal-to-noise ratio in dendrites, where neurons receive signals from hundreds or thousands of other neurons. Thus, the right signals are amplified and irrelevant ones are suppressed. They attune neurons to make perceptual discriminations quickly and accurately and to make the correct decision.

When dopamine is stimulated by a stimulant drug, more neuromodulating molecules are discharged into the fluid around certain neurons. Changes within the sending and target neurons make it easier for them to synchronize; that means that the presynaptic neuron sends a stronger signal across its synapses and the postsynaptic neuron is more likely to respond. Mental processes become faster and more efficient and an effective neural network is quicker to form.

Stimulants improve mental speed by activating natural processes. There are other ways to enhance the speed and accuracy of mental processing, like exercise, meditation and prayer and, of course, a good night's rest. Such benevolent activities increase neuromodulators like dopamine. They are at higher levels when one is well-rested and alert, when one is in good spirits, and at certain times of the day. Natural stimulants like tea and coffee also increase the activity of dopamine. Sexual arousal increases it. Sexual satisfaction brings it down and you can have a nice, relaxing sleep.

Mental processing speed is a fundamental measure of brain health and integrity. Children and adults with ADD tend to have slower processing speed and it gets a bit faster after they take a stimulant. Many other conditions can cause one's mind to operate slowly; if you have a fever, or are sleep-deprived, or stressed; if you drink alcohol or take sedatives or opioids. The speed with which brain can process information is also lower in patients with mental disorders, including schizophrenia, bipolar disorder, depression and anxiety. Mental speed tends to be faster in people who are more intelligent, but mental speed and intelligence are not the same thing. Some very smart people are ponderous thinkers. Mental speed gradually declines as we age; it is attributable to the gradual loss of the neurons that produce dopamine, among other things. Mental speed goes down even more sharply in old people who are not healthy.

Runella's processing speed increased when she took Ritalin, but she was still on the low side of normal. The improvement was enough for her to do better on the LSAT and she got into law school. I deserve all the credit for giving our fair state yet one more lawyer.[†]

In the studies we did, patients with ADD have consistently slower reaction times than normal individuals in simple and complex cognitive tasks. When we gave them a test dose of Ritalin, their speed improved. Ritalin increased reaction time in ADD patients by 10% and Adderall, 15%. However, their mental speed did not increase to normal levels. There are limits what a drug can do, even mighty amphetamine; the limits are set by our individual biology.

When normal, healthy people are given a stimulant their mental processing speed also increases, by about the same amount. Think of what you could accomplish if your every thought and action were 10% faster, or 15%. You could solve the Necker cube in 108 seconds. It would give you an extra hour every day.

Would that were true. There is no reason to believe that the mental speed effect of amphetamine is sustained in normal, healthy people, as it is in patients with ADD or brain injury. A healthy brain regulates the speed with which it operates. It doesn't like too much speed. Or too much anything.

[†] She devoted her career to family law, a singularly unremunerative but estimable branch of the profession, advocating for abused women and children.

27. MEMORY

Stimulants are supposed to be cognitive enhancers and they are, in patients. In normal, healthy individuals, they also improve cognitive functions, but only when low doses are used and only over the short-term. Nevertheless, that 2008 paper in Nature suggested that stimulants enhance memory. Well, do they?

> Gwenn was 68 years old and healthy. Her mother had had Alzheimer's disease, and she was worrying that she might be getting it, too. *I am so forgetful, she said. I keep missing appointments and dates. My children tell me I repeat myself...*

Gwenn did, indeed, have memory deficits when we tested her and she had neurological soft signs suggestive of incipient dementia. After the workup, she was a candidate for one of several drugs that we give to patients with early Alzheimer's. That would ordinarily be Aricept or a similar drug. However, her son-in-law was a physician, and suggested we try Ritalin first. She had a delicate stomach and probably wouldn't tolerate Aricept, which causes GI distress in a lot of patients. The son-in-law was a young fellow, but I am old enough to remember when Dexedrine was routinely given to patients with early dementia. She had never had high blood pressure or heart problems. So, she tried 5 mg of Ritalin. She felt more positive and energetic on the drug but her memory scores didn't improve at all.[*]

> Charles was 29 and was in a motorcycle accident three years prior. He had a traumatic brain injury and a cardiac arrest in the emergency room, with the likelihood of additional brain damage. He was

---

[*] If we had given her cholinesterase inhibitor, Aricept (donepezil), the effect would have been the same. Dementia drugs like Aricept improve energy and attention but not memory.

hospitalized for several weeks and was in rehab for months. He made a good recovery and was even able to return to work. Then he decided to go back to school. He started taking courses at the community college but had problems remembering, even when he went over the material several times.

Charles was a healthy young man and his examination was normal, aside from a lot of scars from the accident. Nevertheless, he had persistent cognitive deficits from the brain injury, especially memory. We gave him a test dose of Ritalin and his scores on tests of memory, attention and processing speed improved. We prescribed a stimulant medication and he was able to do well in school. After a year on Ritalin, he stopped taking the drug, but his memory problems returned. He resumed the drug and went on to graduate.

In some clinical circumstances, amphetamines improve memory. In others, they don't. You have to take it one patient at a time.

Brandon knew that amphetamine improved memory. *I can't say from personal experience but one of my clients told me he could never remember what teachers said in class. When he took Adderall, he could.*

Brandon didn't know I had written a paper in 1986, with two colleagues, that reported improved memory in ADD children who were given Ritalin. The improvement was not correlated with improved attention. In other words, the kids remembered better but not because they were paying attention better. We also reported that stimulants didn't necessarily improve the acquisition of memories (encoding) but, rather the storage of memories (consolidation). What the children learned, they remembered.[62]

It is now well-established that stimulants improve memory

consolidation; taking a stimulant lets you hold onto memories better and longer. It's not because people attend better, which was probably the case for Brandon's client. If you attend to something, you are acquiring it, or encoding it. Consolidation is a different process entirely. It takes a memory that had been encoded and puts it into storage. Stimulants improve memory storage independent of their effects on attention and encoding. They improve storage even if the drug is given *after* the memory is acquired. Stimulants enhance the storage of memories. But is it only a laboratory finding or is it clinically meaningful?

It was meaningful for Charles, and the effect was sustained. When he went off Ritalin, memory problems returned. In his case, the memory effect made a difference. Not for Gwenn. With Ritalin she felt more alert and had more energy, but her memory didn't improve at all. Comparing Charles' response to Gwenn's underscores the fact that stimulant effects depend on the patient and what their pathology is. In Alzheimer's disease new memories are not encoded; there is nothing to consolidate.[63]

In ADD patients, it takes a full neurocognitive battery and statistical analysis to distinguish drug effects on memory from those on attention. There's no point to doing that; the memory effect is statistically significant but clinically meaningless. In experimental subjects, stimulants improve memory consolidation, but the studies are short-term and have never been done in habitual users. There is no reason to believe that stimulants improve the memory of normal people over the long-term. In fact, amphetamine addicts develop persistent deficits in memory.

In real life, a stimulant may let a normal, healthy person hold onto new facts for a few days. College students appreciate that when they cram for an exam. They will remember better if they use a low dose and get a good night's rest before the exam. Unfortunately, they usually do neither. High stimulant doses combined with sleep deprivation tend to impair one's memory. That may explain why college students who use stimulants as study aids don't get better grades than students who don't.

Most of the memory problems that people complain of are not consolidation problems at all. Forgetfulness is part of the human condition, but it is usually an encoding problem; that is, you never aquire the memory. You set down your keys or your iPhone and forget where you left them. You go into a room and forget why you went there. The problem is that you didn't attend to where you put your keys or why you went upstairs to the bedroom, so you never encoded the memory. Theoretically, stimulants ought to help you attend to such things; they are more likely to make you hyperfocus on something else.

You are introduced to someone and take up a conversation, but then you forget their name. The word for it is *proactive inhibition*; the fascinating conversation you enjoyed after the introduction overwrote your memory of their name before it could be consolidated. Or, you can't remember the right word, or the name of someone you know well. That is *dysnomia*, a normal problem that people begin to notice in their 50s (and not a harbinger of Alzheimer's disease). These are universal problems, and my patients tell me they are signs of failing memory. They are not. They are attention problems.

If stimulants were indeed cognitive enhancers for the population at large, we would know by now. The millions of non-ADD adults who take Adderall and similar nostrums would be so smart the rest of us would notice. Have you noticed?

28. SMART DRUGS

Shay was a junior in High School. Her GPA was 3.5 and 4.5, weighted. A weighted GPA credits the student for taking advanced courses, and some kids manage 6.0 or higher. Her father brought her to see me. He was an IT entrepreneur with a prosperous business. He said, *I don't know if she is ADD, but she is not serious enough about her studies and I think a stimulant would make that better...*

A drug that improves attention, mental processing speed and memory should make you smarter. Stimulants do. A lot of studies have examined the question, and the consensus is that stimulant treatment in children with ADD improves their performance on IQ tests. The kids get smarter. So, stimulants are smart drugs.

Not so fast. This is what really happens: ADD kids have cognitive weaknesses that interfere with their performance on IQ tests. Stimulants improve those weaknesses and enable children to perform to their potential. They don't increase their potential or expand their intelligence.

Stimulants don't improve IQ test scores in people who aren't cognitively impaired in the first place. Neither do they make them smarter. That's not what people say, of course. Amphetamines are *cognitive-enhancement technologies*. They enhance your cognitive powers They are *smart drugs*, just like centrophenoxine, piracetam, ginkgo, ketamine, LSD and psilocybin, phosphatidylserine, fish oil, orgone boxes, jellyfish extract, and testicle transplants from baboons. In years past, alcohol, cannabis and opium were promoted for their mind-expanding powers. Periodically, a new substance is added to the list. In lean years, there are new concoctions of the old ones.

Take a breath. If a clever scientist were to develop a drug that made us smarter, or that alleviated normal ageing-related cognitive decline, don't you think her name would be sung from the rooftops? When a drug really works – as Ozempic does for weight loss – the word gets around real fast. Your family doc will give it to you. Insurance will cover it. There would be shortages. And counterfeit versions.

Yet educated men and women say that *They would feel pressure to give cognition-enhancing drugs to their children if other children at school were taking them.*

Shay didn't have attention or processing speed problems that prevented her from reaching her potential. But her father believed that a stimulant would give her a short-term burst of mental energy. *She does poorly on the SATs*, he said. In fact, her SAT scores were well above average. They just weren't as stratospheric as he wanted them to be. *At least she should take a dose before she takes the SAT.*

Shay's father was probably impressed by the many other students at her elite high school who were taking Adderall or Ritalin. They were no more ADD than Shay was. They just wanted better grades to get into an elite college. Why give them an unfair advantage? *My friend gave his son Adderall and he scored a hundred points higher on the SAT.*

For every child like that – if the story were true – I can cite another kid who scored a hundred points *lower*. Someone should do a study: compare the effects of Adderall on the SAT compared to a good night's sleep, a nutritious breakfast and a home environment that promoted confidence rather than anxiety.

Stimulants are cognitive enhancers because they convey an additional measure of mental energy; several of the characters we have met here testify to how useful they are. But the principal is this: that additional burst of mental energy has more meaningful effects in people who are cognitively impaired to begin with. In people who aren't impaired, stimulant effects are at best short-term and at worst unpredictable. They don't have reliable, long-term positive effects on memory, attention, executive functions, creativity or test scores.[64]

> Maxwell was a fourth-year student at a prestigious medical school. His grades were stellar, but his future depended on performance on part two of the medical boards. A score of 35 meant that he would get the residency that he wanted – one of the top training programs in the country. He had three months off from school to prepare for part two, but he could never score higher than 33 on pre-tests.
>
> He had been taking Adderall since college and was still on it as he prepared for the big test. When he told me about his problem, I told him to stop taking Adderall. I explained why. He stopped the drug. His pre-tests promptly improved and he made it to 35.

Maxwell's experience illustrates the INVERTED-U THEORY, proposed in 1908 by psychologists Robert Yerkes and John DODSON. Low doses of a stimulant improve cognitive performance and higher doses impair it.

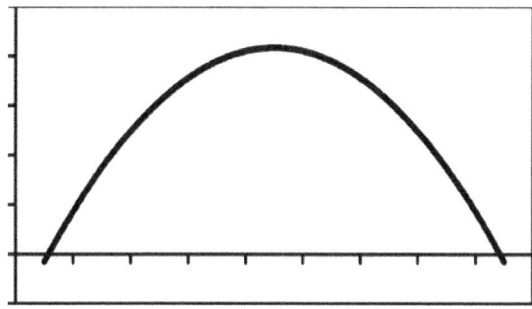

For Dobson and Yerkes, the stimulant in question was an electric shock. Mice had to learn to run into a white box and if they ventured into the black box they got a shock. How fast they learned to avoid the black box was related to the strength of the shock. Shocks of medium intensity made them learn faster; small shocks and strong shocks impaired learning. In subsequent years, the inverted U was explained in terms of arousal. The medium shocks put the mice into a state of optimal arousal, which enhanced learning. Neither too much arousal nor too little were good at all.

The Dobson-Yerkes theory has been elevated over time into a psychological law. Inventive psychologists have applied it to stress, anxiety, weight dissatisfaction and challenging events during childhood; too little or too much is bad, but *this porridge is just right*.

In 1977, my two old friends, Robert Sprague and Eleanor Sleator, demonstrated an inverted U for ADD children treated with Ritalin. A low dose (0.3 mg/kg, or 10 mg for a 75 pound child) improved kids' test performance while a higher dose (20 mg) made the children perform worse. The study affirmed the inverted U effect of Ritalin on cognition. However, there was no such effect on hyperactivity. The higher dose was better than the low dose for making the children behave.[65]

Test performance is a pretty good measure of intelligence, but it isn't all there is to it. Creativity is not something that tests don't measure very well. Colin tested his creativity by doing math proofs.

> Colin had been on Ritalin since grade school. He was ADD and dyslexic, but he did well enough with medication and accommodations to make it to a fine college in our neighborhood. He was a brilliant kid in spite of his disability and did especially well in math. He majored in math and physics and made straight As, but he couldn't pass his humanities courses without Ritalin. I had known Colin for years but when he was in his second year at college we had an interesting conversation.

Colin was taking a moderate dose of long-acting methylphenidate, but only two days a week when he had his general-Ed classes, or when he had to read something or write a paper. *It's amazing,* He said. *It actually helps me to read, just like it did when I was in Middle School. But if I take it, I can't do math. I have a proof to do, and I can't get a handle. The next day, when the stuff is out of my body, the proof comes to me just like that.*

Colin wanted a refill for his medication but he also wanted an explanation. At the time, I was at a loss. I could only tell him that the cognitive effects of stimulants are different in different people. Stimulants don't ordinarily improve a reading disability, but about half of dyslexics also have ADD, so treating them with a stimulant helps them to focus better and struggle through reading. He told me that he knew that but he didn't understand why the drug would impair math.

Colin was my patient more than 30 years ago. At the time, our experience with ADD in adults was limited. In ADD children, stimulant effects are predictable. It's because the cognitive challenges they face are limited. Schoolwork tends to be laborious and a bit dull. Stimulants are good for that.

ADD adults have to deal with a wider variety of challenges, many of which involve flexibility, strategic planning and creativity. Stimulants are more likely to impair performance in such activities.

Generating a proof in higher math is a creative process. In Colin, the Ritalin that allowed him to overcome dyslexia impeded his ability to be creative in math. The smart drug made him smarter in one domain but not another.

Solving a proof in higher math requires flexibility, strategic planning and creativity. Flexibility means more than switching from one task to another and then back again. It is the essence of creativity which is, by definition, growing something new and different. The creative process takes up empty spaces in one's mind. Stimulant drugs keep those empty spaces closed.[66]

Stimulants might make a creative person more productive because she is more alert and has more energy in her head. They may even help her get stuff done 10% faster. But they may also freeze her cognitive flexibility. What she gets done during that 90% won't be so creative at all.[67]

Stimulant drugs don't make people smarter. They make people *feel* smarter. For some people, that's enough.

29. PERSONAL USE (AGAIN)

Psychostimulants *are* smart drugs. They are the only molecules that reliably improve attention, memory and psychomotor speed.[68] In patients, they are quite effective over the long-term. In normal, healthy people, they have small, short-term effects. They exercise their beneficial effects by generating mental energy and enhancing the efficiency of neuronal communication. They affect the regulatory apparatus of the brain, the central executive.

If the cognitive effects of amphetamines in normal people are so limited, why do so many normal people like to take them?

Not a hard question. Stimulants make you feel good. They are energy drugs and everyone would like a bit more energy. They also enhance one's sense of well-being, especially when one is doing something that is important but mildly disagreeable. Stimulants improve one's attention to dull, boring tasks because such tasks are effortful and mildly disagreeable.

Stimulants are popular because the symptoms of ADD are ubiquitous. We can't always muster the concentration needed to get stuff done. Relying on stimulants for that extra burst of energy can become a habit.

Some more reasons:

- Mild, subclinical ADD afflicts one person in seven. Mild, subclinical learning disabilities are equally common. From time to time, such mild problems become problematic.
- Normal, healthy ageing is associated with gradual decline in energy, attention, psychomotor speed and memory. Not all of us want to take it lying down, although a nice nap can be stimulating, too.

- Fatigue is one of the commonest complaints patients make to their doctors. Remember: role overload.
- When Benzedrine was first marketed in 1933, Smith, Klein & French suggested it was good for 'minor depression'. How many normal, healthy people are minorly depressed? Or worry too much?

I would give you yet another, but I don't want to sound like a cynic. Well... Two double lattés a day cost $400 a month. Even more if you like lavender oat-milk chai lattés. Your co-pay for a month of Adderall is $20 and you don't have to walk around all day carrying a cup.

More than 11 million Americans take prescription stimulants, and only a small fraction of them are ADD children grown up. The vast majority are more-or-less normal people who need a little help. What's wrong with that? Nothing, it seems, as long as one knows what he or she is doing and does it carefully.

During the 20th century, there was a consensus that mind-altering drugs were not good and mostly dangerous. Their use should be discouraged if not suppressed. Citizens of the 21st century have come to a different conclusion. Forbidden drugs might not be so bad after all. They may even be useful. In any event, mentally competent adults should be allowed to decide for themselves.

Like most children of the sixties, I am a libertarian at heart. But my life since then has been that of a physician who treats real people. I know what's good and what's bad, even when patients disagree. Most of them are mentally competent, but they don't know what I know.

I know that the ready availability of amphetamines in ADD World is neither good nor bad. It is both, depending. Most so-called ADDs are something else, as we have seen; some of them can be treated with stimulants and for others, it's a bad choice. Even real ADDs are a diverse group. They have similar symptoms but there are different reasons why those symptoms occur, and not every real ADD needs a stimulant.

Amphetamines are good or bad, depending on the person, why he takes the drug and how she takes it. They are not dangerous drugs, but useful treatments, when they are used right. To do right, you providers need to know why you are prescribing amphetamine. You patients need to know why you are taking it. You both need to know what amphetamines do and how they do it, and also what they don't do.

Stimulants are safe when they aren't used too much. Stimulants are safe for children but they're not so good for fetuses or little babies. They aren't so good for people at cardiovascular risk. If you are taking other drugs, stimulants may augment their beneficial effects or cause them to have toxic effects.

Stimulants may alleviate ADD symptoms in patients with chronic mental illness. But then, there is the problem of drug interactions. Also, most mental illnesses are cardiovascular risk factors in their own right.

I wish stimulants worked better for brain-fog, but sometimes they have marvelous effects.

Stimulants are good for fatigue and minor depression. But there are a lot of other ways to treat fatigue and minor depression that are risk-free.

Maybe low dose stimulants are good for your brain, though I doubt it. Even if they are, I think that green tea, olive oil and garlic are better.

Stimulants are good for many of the problems that old people have. Like antidepressants, they may delay brain ageing or the onset of ageing-related dementia. Old people need ten hours of good sleep, though, so you don't want a drug that interferes with sleep. In fact, ageing is accelerated in people who don't sleep well. And then, there are those extra few pulse beats per minute, and a few millimeters of Mercury in blood pressure – they add up, over the years.

The likelihood of heart attack or stroke is low in a healthy young person who takes low doses of amphetamine. It's not so low in older people. Amphetamine use – in whatever dose – has to be considered a cardiovascular risk factor. Amphetamines may not be so risky as smoking, diabetes, high blood pressure, cholesterol or obesity, but maybe they are. We shall find out before long – those eleven million American adults are lab rats who will answer the question.

Warning that prescription amphetamines are addicting drugs is technically true, but the information has no impact on the people who take low doses under supervision. Amphetamine addiction causes heart attack, psychosis and dementia, but I am not into fearmongering here. Nevertheless, regular use, even under medical supervision, can turn into a habit and habits are not always easy to control. Habitual users are prone to irritability and anger, obsessiveness and depression. Their proposed solution is a higher dose. The good thing about medical supervision is that we can catch that before it gets out of hand. Real supervision, that is, not some incognito 'provider' on Zoom.

Speaking as a not-so-libertarian physician who has treated patients for more than 50 years, a whole lot of amphetamines spread across the population makes me uneasy. It suggests to me that medical supervision is not as careful as it should be. It means that uncommon or mild side effects will be amplified by the sheer fact of widespread use. It also means more pills that will be diverted. Protecting the public health means limiting the availability of amphetamines. Increasing their availability only increases the occurrence of baleful effects.

To individuals, of course, the public health is less important than their immediate need. To some, the problem of availability is that there's not enough. *That stupid doctor won't give me a prescription. I'm on 30 migs of Adderall three times a day but I still can't focus. This ADD is killing me.*

NOTES

1, page 1. *Ten million American adults take stimulant drugs.*

This is what the medical journals say: US prevalence rates for ADHD in children range around 6.5%. Estimates for adults vary widely across studies, but average around 2.5–3.4%. Meta-analyses cite estimates ranging between 1.4 and 3.6%.(Franke et al., 2018)

Now, the data:

- 9.5%, more than seven million US kids, diagnosed with ADD.
- 62% of ADD children taking medication, more than three million kids.
- 4.5%, more than 11 million US adults used stimulants for ADD.

The numbers are from 2016 and are higher now. There weren't amphetamine shortages in 2016. Stimulants were prescribed to 3.6% of the US population in 2016 and 4.1% in 2021, a 14% increase. (Danielson, 2023)

The prevalence of ADD is not like the prevalence of HIV infection or breast cancer or pregnancy. The diagnosis is analog, not digital. Like hypertension, diabetes and hyperlipidemia, it is possible to have just a little bit of the disorder, or a whole lot. Like cholesterol, what represents an abnormal state can change as physicians' opinions about the condition change. The prevalence of ADD is not a number that describes how many people have the condition, but rather, how many people are thought to have the condition. Or how many think they have the condition.

PREVALENCE IN CHILDREN

The numbers are all over the place, as you might expect of a condition whose borders are fuzzy, insofar as they exist at all.

In the past, ADD was uncommon: in 1966, fewer than 1% of children in England (Rutter & Graham, 1966) and in 1973, 1-2% of Swedish schoolchildren.(Blythe, 1979) Even in those days, there were foreshadowings. In 1971, Paul Wender estimated that the "Hyperkinetic reaction of childhood" (DSM2) afflicted 5-10% of all schoolchildren. (Wender, 1971) Wender was an esteemed prominent and prolific psychiatrist who had done seminal research on a number of subjects. His ideas about ADD were supported by prominent child psychiatrists in the US; American pediatricians and British psychiatrists were dubious.

Wender's estimates were prescient. Recent reviews suggest that the global prevalence of ADHD is between 2% and 7%, with an average around 5%. But an additional 5% have difficulties with overactivity, inattention, and impulsivity that are just under the threshold to meet the diagnostic criteria for ADHD. (Wilens et al., 2008) (Willcutt, 2012) (Sayal et al., 2018) (Song et al., 2019) The prevalence of ADD around the world ranges from less than 1% in some studies (Polanczyk et al., 2007) to 16% in Rochester, Minnesota, home of the Mayo Clinic. (Barbaresi et al., 2002) In my state, the ADHD prevalence rate is 15.5%. (Rowland et al., 2015)

In the face of such confusion, I shall rely on these two surveys: the 2007 National Health Interview Survey reported that the US lifetime prevalence of clinically diagnosed ADD among 4- to 17-year-olds was 9.5%, about 5.4 million children. In 2016, the National Survey of Children's Health, a nationally representative, cross-sectional survey of parents regarding their children's health, estimated that 6.1 million U.S. children 2-17 years of age (9.4%) had an ADHD diagnosis. (Danielson et al., 2018) There were 77 million children in the USA in 2020. If 9.5% is a sound estimate, more than seven million US kids are ADD. More than half are taking stimulants.

During the nineteen-seventies, the prescription of stimulants to schoolchildren increased threefold. In 1973, the first survey of medications for hyperactive children reported that 1.7% of schoolchildren in Baltimore were treated with stimulants. (Safer

& Krager, 1983). By 1987, no fewer than 6% of all public elementary school students in Baltimore County were receiving the drugs.(Safer & Krager, 1988) In the next few years, the practice spread to the secondary schools, and girls began to be treated in ever-greater numbers (Safer & Krager, 1994). In 2016, the National Survey of Children's Health reported that 62% of ADD children were taking medication, that is, more than three million kids.

Whatever the precise number – and precision is never going to characterize research on this topic -- ADD is the most common cognitive disorder in the population at large. And it's not just America anymore. Stimulant prescription for ADD is increasing in Canada, Western Europe, Asia and Australia. (Safer & Zito, 2010) (Raman et al., 2018)

ADULTS

Speaking of precision: adult ADD occurs either in 1% or 7% of Americans, or so they say. (Simon et al., 2009) (Katzman et al., 2017). The number you encounter in most medical papers is around 2.5% but when ADD is 'defined broadly' the rate goes up to 16.4%. (Faraone & Biederman, 2005)

In 2014, stimulant prescription for adults exceeded, for the first time, prescriptions for children. (Safer, 2016) Stimulant prescription for adults has increased since then. In 2011, 0.3% of all prescriptions written for adults were for stimulants; in 2019, it was 1.5% of all prescriptions, a fivefold increase in 8 years. (Rasmussen, 2008) A national survey in 2016 found that about 6.6% of US adults (16 million) used prescription stimulants in the preceding year; 4.5% (or 11 million) used prescription stimulants appropriately, without misuse; 2.1% (or 5 million) misused prescription stimulants at least once; and 0.2% (or 0.4 million) were stimulant abusers. (Compton et al., 2018) ('Misuse' means they used stimulants without medical supervision. 'Abuse' means using stimulants in potentially harmful way and includes addiction.) The National Center for Drug Abuse Statistics, however, reported that 9% of US adults misused or abused prescription stimulants in 2019. (http://drugabusestatistics.org/)

ADD rates in adults don't include the number who borrow stimulants from friends (or from their children) or who buy stimulants on the internet. For example, 10-20% of college students (and medical students) use stimulants without a prescription. (McCabe et al., 2005) (Arria et al., 2008) (Teter et al., 2006) (Finger et al., 2013) (Webb et al., 2013) The number of adults who take stimulants without medical supervision is probably as high as the number who manage to wheedle a prescription.

2, p1. *ADD is a neurodevelopmental disorder.*

According to the DSM-5-tr, the most recent dictionary of psychiatric disorders, "ADHD is a neurodevelopmental disorder defined by impairing levels of inattention, disorganization, and/or hyperactivity-impulsivity. Inattention and disorganization entail inability to stay on task, seeming not to listen, and losing materials necessary for tasks, at levels that are inconsistent with age or developmental level. Hyperactivity-impulsivity entails overactivity, fidgeting, inability to stay seated, intruding into other people's activities, and inability to wait— symptoms that are excessive for age or developmental level." (American Psychiatric Association, 2022)

The DSM-5-tr lists three presentations of ADHD: Predominantly Inattentive, Hyperactive-Impulsive and Combined. The diagnostic criteria require symptoms and/or behaviors to have persisted for at least 6 months in at least 2 settings (e.g., school, home, church). Symptoms must have negatively impacted academic, social, and/or occupational functioning. In patients younger than 17, at least 6 symptoms are necessary; in those aged 17 and older, at least 5 symptoms are necessary.

Inattentive Type
• Displays poor listening skills.

• Loses and/or misplaces items needed to complete activities or tasks.
• Sidetracked by external or unimportant stimuli.
• Forgets daily activities.
• Diminished attention span.
• Lacks ability to complete schoolwork and other assignments or to follow instructions.
• Avoids or is disinclined to begin homework or activities requiring concentration.
• Fails to focus on details and/or makes thoughtless mistakes in schoolwork or assignments.

Hyperactive/Impulsive Type
Hyperactive Symptoms:
• Squirms when seated or fidgets with feet/hands.
• Marked restlessness that is difficult to control.
• Appears to be driven by "a motor" or is often "on the go".
• Lacks ability to play and engage in leisure activities in a quiet manner.
• Incapable of staying seated in class.
• Overly talkative.

Impulsive Symptoms:
• Difficulty waiting turn.
• Interrupts or intrudes into conversations and activities of others.
• Impulsively blurts out answers before questions completed.

Additional Requirements for Diagnosis
• Symptoms must be present prior to age 12 years.
• Symptoms not better accounted for by a different psychiatric disorder (e.g., mood disorder, anxiety disorder) and do not occur exclusively during a psychotic disorder (e.g., schizophrenia).
• Symptoms not exclusively a manifestation of oppositional

behavior.

"Several of the symptoms must have been present prior to age 12. This generally requires corroboration by a parent or some other informant. It is important to note that the presence of significant impairment in at least two major settings of the person's life is central to the diagnosis of ADHD. Examples of impairment include losing a job because of ADHD symptoms, experiencing excessive conflict and distress in a marriage, getting into financial trouble because of impulsive spending, failure to pay bills in a timely manner or being put on academic probation in college due to failing grades. If the individual exhibits a number of ADHD symptoms, but they do not cause significant impairment, s/he may not meet the criteria to be diagnosed with ADHD as a clinical disorder.

"In making the diagnosis, adults should have at least five of the symptoms present. These symptoms can change over time, so adults may fit different presentations from when they were children."

The definition is said to be an example of circular logic: "if A then B, and if B then A." If an individual has attention deficit hyperactivity disorder it is because he is inattentive, disorganized and hyperactive-impulsive, and if an individual is inattentive, disorganized and hyperactive-impulsive it is because he has attention deficit hyperactivity disorder. (Tait, 2009) (Koutsoklenis & Honkasilta, 2023)

3, p 4. ADHD sounds like sneezing:

ADHD is the correct but clumsy acronym, Attention Deficit/Hyperactivity Disorder. It used to be just Attention Deficit Disorder, or ADD. I'm stuck with ADD, and for good reason. Think of all the acronyms you know. How many have an H? Don't say "What about OTOH?" No one *says* "OTOH". It's text-speak. Think of the acronyms we say as if they were words, like OC, PDF, ATM, DNA, SUV, USA, ASAP, SOS, IQ, TGIF,

RSVP, MD, GOP, HR, MBA, AM & PM, RADAR, FBI... No aitches at all.

BTW, ADDerall isn't ADHDerall.

These are the names our favorite neurodevelopmental disorder has had over the ages:
- Minimal brain damage (MBD) (Strauss & Lehtinen, 1947)
- Hyperkinetic impulse disorder (Laufer et al., 1957)
- Minimal cerebral dysfunction (Bax & MacKeith, 1963)
- Minimal brain dysfunction (MBD) (Wender, 1971)
- Hyperkinetic reaction of childhood (DSM-II, 1968)
- Attention deficit disorder: with and without hyperactivity (ADD) (DSM-III, 1980)
- Attention deficit hyperactivity disorder (ADHD) (DSM-III-R, 1987, ff.)

In 1942, the child psychiatrist, Lauretta Bender, described MBD kids as 'hyperkinetic'. It means hyperactive.

4, p8. *Neurological soft signs and minor physical anomalies.*

Minor physical anomalies (MPAs) are slight physical deviations that have no serious medical or cosmetic significance but suggest that something was amiss early in a child's embryological development. The list of MPAs includes multiple hair whorls, electric hair, floppy or low set ears, widely spaced eyes and epicanthal folds, high arched palate, geographic tongue, transverse palmar crease, curved fifth finger, third toe longer than the second and a big gap between the first and second toes. A normal person might have one or two such MPAs, a child with dyslexia or ADD four or five, an autistic child five or six and a child with Down syndrome eight or ten.

A large number of genes regulate head, face and brain development, so physical anomalies suggest a genetic aberration, severe ones in children with intellectual disability and mild ones in children with learning disabilities and ADD. Anomalies may also be related to prenatal infection or fetal exposure to alcohol or certain drugs. (Ozgen et al., 2008)

Developmental disorders are also associated with neurological softs signs. Soft signs, by definition, are not hard, that is, they don't refer to a cerebral location or indicate a specific lesion or disease. They indicate diffuse CNS dysfunction or dysmaturation. They are like physical anomalies, insignificant in their own right, but meaningful when they occur in strength or number, or when they support a diagnosis already suspected. Neurological soft signs include choreiform movements, abnormalities of muscle tone, asymmetric reflexes, problems with rapid alternating movements and finger-thumb opposition, overflow movements, sequencing difficulties, impersistence, right-left confusion, difficulties with stereognosis or graphesthesia, extinction in response to double simultaneous stimulation, gait imbalance (tandem walk) and an impaired stance with eyes closed. (Gillberg & Kadesjö, 2003)

Neurological soft signs and MPAs have a quantitative association with developmental disorders. Patients with ADHD or LD have a few more than normal controls, and patients with autism have more than they do. Schizophrenics have more than their first degree relatives who, in turn, have more than normal controls. (C. T. Gualtieri et al., 1982) (Neelam et al., 2011) (Varambally et al., 2012)

5, p10. *The myelination of frontal neurons is not completed until the fifth decade.*

Myelin is a rubbery substance that coats nerve fibers, axons and dendrites. It enables the transmission of nervous impulses with greater speed and efficiency down the dendrites to the neuronal cell body and away from the neuron body on the axons. An infant's brain is only partially myelinated and most of the brain is myelinated by age 20. The prefrontal cortex is among the last brain regions to be completely myelinated, usually by age 50 or so. It's why old people have good judgment and deep wells of wisdom, in contrast to young people, who don't. (Yakovlev, 1962) (Yakovlev, 1967) (Benes et al., 1994)

6, p12. *A lot of people are going to be ADD*

Studies from 1958 to 2008 showed that about a third of all children are overactive, fidgety or distractible. In the Isle of Wight study, 75% of the dull children were rated by teachers as inattentive, but 30-50% of the brighter children were also so described. (Wortis, 1984) Teachers rated 29% of 9- to 12-year-olds as restless or fidgety and 33% had poor concentration. Psychiatrists interviewed the children and thought that 51% were fidgety. (Graham & Rutter, 1968) In a Chicago survey in 1958, a survey of 482 mothers reported that 49% of their children were overactive and 30% were restless. (Lapouse & Monk, 1958) More recent surveys of parents and teachers indicate that kids are as obstreperous as they ever were. What has changed is, now they are 'diagnosed'.(Safer, 2018) The prevalence of the ADD diagnosis grew as soon as people realized it was there.

7, p 14. *We have yet to discover negative long-term effects.*

The Adderall-Ritalin family of stimulant drugs also includes MDMA, methamphetamine and cocaine, and now 'designer drugs' that have stimulant-like effects. Such drugs are highly addictive and clearly dangerous. Some are neurotoxic – they injure brain cells – or they cause heart attack and sudden death. It is not appropriate, however, to compare clinical use of stimulants to what happens to methamphetamine and cocaine addicts. Meth is more potent and stays longer in the brain; cocaine affects different molecules in the brain. The doses addicts use are at least ten times higher than therapeutic doses and often fifty or a hundred times higher.

8, p14. *Motor and phonic tics.*

Tics are sudden eruptions of motor or phonic activity, such as facial grimaces, shrugs, twitches, throat-clearing, shouts, sometimes even dirty words (coprolalia). They are frequent concomitants of normal development – ten per cent of 10-year-old boys have motor or phonic tics. Tics can be annoying or even painful, but they are innocent events, and when a stimulant causes tics it doesn't mean the things will last forever. They disappear when the dose is lowered or when the drug is stopped, although it may take a while. Some children find tics embarrassing but most kids don't even notice. Sometimes, parents don't even notice. Tics rarely occur when adults take stimulants.

9, p14. *The effects are apparent an hour after the child gets a test dose.*

Immediate-release formulations of methylphenidate and amphetamine reach peak levels in 45-60 minutes. It our clinics, it is customary to start stimulant treatment with a 'test dose' of Ritalin (0.3 mg/kg in children, 15-20 mg in adults) or Adderall (0.2 mg/kgm in children, 10-15 mg in adults). The patient goes off for lunch and returns an hour later, when we re-test and measure effects on heart rate and blood pressure. It's a good way to discover if the drug is going to be helpful or if it will have side effects. Sometimes tics will start after only one dose (see 8). Sometimes a patient will have a catastrophic reaction and return in tears. It is always an opportunity to educate the patient, or parents, about stimulant drugs; to get a good idea what dose may be right; and to assure ourselves that we are doing the right thing. After the test dose, we give the patient a 2 week supply of Ritalin and (in older kids and adults) a 2 week supply of Adderall, to compare. There is simply no way to predict which drug the patient will prefer.

10, p16. *The first controlled clinical trial was published in 1967.*

"Fifty-two children with learning problems were treated with dextroamphetamine sulfate and a matched placebo in a double-blind, crossover design over a two-month period. Significant improvement in teacher ratings of behavior was demonstrated under the active drug condition. A battery of performance tests derived from an earlier factor-analytic study showed reliable increases on a factor thought to reflect assertiveness and drive, while a factor primarily measuring intellectual ability was unaffected by the drug.

"The effects in the present study are probably of a motivational nature. Whether direct effects on learning processes such as storage and short-term memory also occur remains to be explored. However, we would surmise that the drug has energized the children, apathetic and discouraged by previous school failure, into making use of abilities available to them. This motivational change is consistent with Bradley's earlier clinical descriptions of changes in the child's interest in surroundings and zest for normal routine activities which had previously been difficult to carry out." (Conners et al., 1967)

11, p17. *What happened to hyperactive children when they were given antipsychotic drugs.*

I got in trouble over this one. Mellaril, an antipsychotic drug, was widely advertised as a safe and effective treatment for ADD kids. Our research group discovered that two-thirds of the kids who took antipsychotic drugs for a period of time developed tardive dyskinesia, a disfiguring and painful movement disorder. In half of those kids, the movement disorder persisted for months or more than a year. (C. T. Gualtieri et al., 1984) I was more than a bit exercised over this and asserted that such drugs had no role in the treatment of ADD. Our research was reported in the national press. Adult psychiatrists got mad at me because they thought I was fueling antipsychotic drug noncompliance in patients with schizophrenia. It precipitated my decline from momentary prominence to well-deserved obscurity, and I have no regrets.

12, p17. *Normal children and normal adults responded just as hyperactive children did.*

"The behavioral, cognitive, and electrophysiological effects of a single dose of dextroamphetamine (0.5 milligram per kilogram of body weight) or placebo was examined in 14 normal prepubertal boys (mean age, 10 years 11 months) in a double-blind study. When amphetamine was given, the group showed a marked decrease in motor activity and reaction time and improved performance on cognitive tests. The similarity of the response observed in normal children to that reported in children with "hyperactivity" or minimal brain dysfunction casts doubt on pathophysiological models of minimal brain dysfunction which assume that children with this syndrome have a clinically specific or "paradoxical" response to stimulants." (Rapoport et al., 1978)

"Methylphenidate was administered to each of 12 adult volunteers in a double-blind, placebo-controlled, crossover study for purposes of comparison with previous studies in hyperactive children. Statistically significant changes occurred only on a minority of measures, but the results were generally in the direction of facilitated performance, reduced physical activity and increased emotional responsivity. As these results are similar to those in hyperactive and normal children, this appears to support the contention that stimulant drug effects in hyperactive children are not paradoxical or atypical." (Aman et al., 1984)

13, p17. *We should have known.*

Evidence for the use of amphetamine for cognitive enhancement dates back decades. For example, "Young male inmates displayed enhancement in physical (strength of grip) and mental performance after amphetamine administration (10, 20, or 30 mg)". (Molitch & Eccles, 1937) Patients with diagnoses ranging from anxiety to schizophrenia experienced an average 8% improvement on an IQ test with 20 mg of amphetamine. (Sargent, 1936) Early articles also report evidence for academic doping. Severe cardiac collapse occurred after excessive amphetamine had been self-administered by one individual who "said the drug was being used to some extent by individuals studying for examinations." (Davies, 1939) Other early reports proclaimed that college students "have great interest in stimulants or 'pep pills' that promise to help them over their academic hurdles" (Flory & Gilbert, 1943) and that "many students have come to cherish this drug as a gift of the Gods, relying upon it to carry them through prolonged periods of cramming for examinations." (Minkowsky, 1939) (Wood et al., 2014a)

"Meanwhile, psychologists quickly established that improvements on intelligence tests were more subjective than real; any gains in performance—typically, in simple tasks requiring persistence—stemmed mainly from amphetamine's ability to increase confidence and initiative rather than actual improvement in mental capacity. These findings did nothing to discourage university students, who evidently did not mind whether amphetamine improved their marks or just made study more bearable." (Wood et al., 2014b)

"The early British studies on amphetamine were mostly careful affairs in university laboratories. Volunteers took a battery of psychological and hand—eye coordination tests. In the majority, amphetamine did not consistently improve performance, though in a few cases—such as the "pursuit meter," a device with a joystick and crosshairs to track a moving target— amphetamine slowed decline in performance. The researchers concluded that the exceptional drug-induced higher scores reflected a subject's attitude toward testing. Because amphetamine users felt more confident and lost interest in tedious tasks less quickly, they maintained effort and did better—just as American psychologists had recently concluded about amphetamine's effect in exams and standardized tests. Yet, in general, amphetamine's boost to performance appeared to be illusory. What Bartlett reported to the FPRC about amphetamines' effect on work capacity applied to most performance measures: 'Individuals were disposed to try to make greater efforts; they thought they were working harder, whereas they were doing exactly the same amount of work.'" (Wood et al., 2014a)

The German Army ran on Pervitin, methamphetamine, which made them more alert. The Japanese army consumed methamphetamine mixed with green tea powder, and so did Japanese workers in armaments and munitions factories. Kamikaze pilots began their terminal fights with a special ceremony, a wreath of flowers and a large intravenous dose of meth. The Allies preferred Benzedrine, an amphetamine not unlike Adderall, especially among bomber pilots, but were ultimately deterred by the effects of the drug, which led to problems with poor judgment, irritability and aggressiveness. The Wehrmacht, who used higher doses of the more potent methamphetamine, ran into problems with depression, psychosis and suicide.

Following the War, amphetamines remained freely available and there were serious epidemics of amphetamine abuse in several countries. In North America, amphetamines were marketed as diet pills; detail men would distribute samples to doctors' offices and office staff took full advantage. It wasn't until 1971 that amphetamines were listed as controlled substances. By that time, the USA had its own epidemic of speed freaks.

The judicious use of Benzedrine in the battle of the North Atlantic illustrates the beneficial effects of low doses on alertness and sustained attention in people who are not ADD. It improved the ability of Sonar operators to detect German submarines. The uncontrolled use of high doses in other spheres of the War illustrates the problems that accrue with high doses. The post-War epidemics showed that when stimulants are freely available, people will take advantage, for reasons that are good and not-so-good.

14, p22. *Personality is the way we are, and we human beings enjoy a lot of it*

This was a dilemma for psychologists who wanted to study personality in a systematic way: where to begin? Gordon Allport, a psychologist at Harvard, decided to begin with the dictionary. Allport and Henry Odbert of Dartmouth College assigned three anonymous people to categorize adjectives from Webster's New International Dictionary and a list of common slang words that referred to the qualities of human beings. (Allport & Odbert, 1936) The three anonymous assistants found 17,953 adjectives in Webster's dictionary that described aspects of the human personality. That was hundred years ago and I'm sure there are more adjectives now. The Urban Dictionary didn't exist in 1924 and Allport didn't know that Neapolitans can describe people with hand gestures and shrugs. Anyway, Allport & Odbert honed the number down to 4504 distinct adjectives to describe human traits.

The three anonymous people didn't just *count* the adjectives, they actually wrote them down, all 17,953 adjectives, among them *wowf, zebrine, smockfaced, smopple, pubigerous* and *looby*. Allport and Odbert threw them out and about 13,000 more, and you can only imagine how the three anonymous people felt about that. The conclusion of this endeavor was to establish that 4504 English adjectives were sufficient to described observable and relatively permanent human traits. (Allport & Odbert, 1936)

In 1943, Raymond Cattell of Harvard University took the list, reduced it to "160 odd" terms and added a few of his own. He wound up with a list of 171 traits. Then he used a new statistical method, factor analysis, to derive 60 "personality clusters or syndromes" plus an additional 7 minor clusters. (R. B. Cattell, 1943) He narrowed it further to 35 terms, and later added a 36th. Then he got it down to 11 or 12 factor solutions. (R. B. Cattell, 1947) That is, human personalities fell into 11 or 12 categories.

In 1947, German-British psychologist, Hans Eysenck of University College London, published his book *Dimensions of Personality*. He proposed that the two most important personality dimensions were "Extraversion" (as opposed to introversion) and "Neuroticism" (opposed to calmness). (H. Eysenck, 1950)

In 1949, Cattell reported that he had found 4 additional factors. He finally published the sixteen factor 16PF Questionnaire, which is still in wide use around the world. (H. E. P. Cattell & Mead, 2008) The 19PF contains 5 global factors (Extraversion/Introversion, High/Low anxiety, Tough-Mindedness/Receptivity, Independence/Accommodation, and Self-Control/Lack of Restraint) and 16 'primary factors' (Warmth, Reasoning, Emotional Stability, Dominance, Liveliness, Consciousness, Boldness, Sensitivity, Vigilance, Abstractedness, Privateness, Apprehension, Openness to Change, Self-Reliance, Perfectionism and Tension).

In the culmination of this extraordinary exercise in adjectival reduction, psychologists have collected data from women and men in all the corners of Earth. Applying ever more clever statistical manipulations, they reduced the number of relevant adjectives to ten, which, in an uncharacteristic burst of colloquialism they call the Big Five:

- Conscientious, as opposed to Careless.
- Agreeable, as opposed to Surly.
- Neurotic, as opposed to Calm.
- Open to experience, as opposed to Narrow-minded.

- Extraverted, as opposed to Introverted.

The Big Five are the five dimensions of personality, five continua or spectra. All of us fall somewhere in between the two poles of each dimension and some of us are at the tips. The Big Five are supposed to contain the basic traits from which every personality is constructed. The traits on each dimension are subject to shadings or gradations, and the combinations and permutations among the five dimensions are virtually infinite. That is about right. Individuals are different, you may have noticed, one from another, and some of us are more different than others.

The personality test you know, one that you may have taken yourself, is the Myers-Briggs Type Indicator. It was invented by a mother-daughter pair in Washington, DC, who had no training in psychology or statistics. They based the test on a misunderstanding of Carl Jung's theory of personality types and proposed four 'preference dichotomies' which are dominant throughout one's life (Extraversion-Introversion, Sensing-Intuition, Thinking-Feeling, and Judging-Perceiving). Unlike the Big Five, whose dimensions contain gradations, the four preferences are dichotomous; individuals are one or the other, all the time, never in between. That, in itself, is a fallacy. It's an odd belief for a test that will generate different results if you take it at different times. The Myers-Briggs exists in a parallel universe, eschewed by well-trained psychologists for its lack of substance or clinical relevance. It is popular among HR officers and some counselors. It gives them something to talk about.

Researchers have tried to relate ADD to personality theory, mostly to the Big Five, which is the prevailing model in American psychology. You can imagine where ADDs fall on the Conscientious/Careless continuum. Conscientiousness is a measure of the degree to which the individual is able to control impulses and delay gratification. (Nigg et al., 2002) (Parker et al., 2004)

ADDs are impulsive. They may be brusque, disinhibited,

thoughtless or socially inappropriate. They score low on the Agreeableness dimension, a measure of getting along with others. (Parker et al., 2004) (Miller et al., 2008) (Miller et al., 2008)

ADDs are excitable. ADDs score high on Neuroticism, which is a measure of emotional stability. (Nigg et al., 2002) (Parker et al., 2004) (Martel et al., 2008) (Miller et al., 2008)

ADDs are sensation-seekers. Extraversion is a measure of sensation seeking. ADDs score high on that. (White, 1999)

The conclusion is that ADD symptoms are reliably associated with personality traits, suggesting (to researchers) "a complex interplay across development." (Knouse et al., 2013) To me, it's not that complicated. It's just describing the same thing in two ways:

Carelessness is a symptom of ADD.
John is careless.
Therefore, John has ADD.

Or:

If one is careless, he is not conscientious.
John is careless.
Therefore, John scores low on the personality trait of conscientiousness.

Don't you love brain science?

15, p23. *I'll let you know.*

The third fact is the prevalence of ADD: almost 10% of children and adults. When a mental disorder is discovered to occur in such high numbers, it means one of two things: either there is something fundamentally wrong with the human race, or we are diagnosing mental disorders in people who have comparatively mild problems. The second explanation is probably right. 10% means you're just one standard deviation out on that bell curve, that is, well within the wide boundaries of normal.

At this point, it will be a good idea to understand the terms we are bandying about as if we knew what they mean. First, a neurodevelopmental disorder. What is that?

Let's drop the neuro- for now. It's just a bit of fluff inserted to make ADD look like brain science. A *developmental disorder* is an aberration in brain development – a condition that deviates from normal brain development and that affects cognitive, emotional, social or motor behavior in an untoward way. Cerebral palsy, intellectual disability and autism are developmental disorders. So is MBD and what I call real ADD.

Developmental disorders are different from developmental *variations*. Variation just means that people are different. Developmental variations are ubiquitous; every brain develops in its individual way and no brain develops in a perfectly normative way in every domain of function. No one's perceptual, cognitive, social, emotional and motor functions are all up to par at every stage of life. Every individual is endowed with strengths and afflicted with weaknesses.

The boundary between developmental disorders and developmental variations is blurry. When is ADD a disorder and when is it just a variation? The answer to the question is the essence of the argument I make in this small book. To understand the answer, let me define three more terms: impairment, disability and handicap.

The failure to exercise the necessary levels of executive control in certain circumstances is an *impairment*. An impairment is a problem in the structure or function of an organ of the body; in this case, the brain, in particular, the brain's Central Executive.

ADD patients and normal people with ADD symptoms have an impairment in their executive faculties. It may be mild or severe, transient, long-lasting or persistent. Not every impairment is disabling.

All three boys – Martin, Felix and Henry -- had an impairment in executive control. In Martin's case, it was caused by perinatal injury. In Felix' case and Henry's, to put it crudely, it was a result of how their brains were wired; they inherited a lot of ADD genes. Technically, an impairment is "any loss or abnormality of psychological, physiological or anatomical structure or function".

Not every impairment is *disabling*. Henry was briefly disabled on two occasions. A disability is a "restriction or lack of ability to perform an activity in the manner or within the range considered normal for a human being". Henry's disability was transient and easily dealt with. It was more than compensated by his many positive qualities. It's a stretch to say he had a disorder. So, too, are most of the children and adults who are said to have ADD.

What makes ADD a disorder in some people is that their impairment results in disability, an inability to do the kinds of things that children of a certain age are expected to do. Felix had a developmental disorder, a disability that was a persistent, life-long problem. He had to make adjustments in the way he did things and he needed intermittent medication treatment. But he lived a happy, productive life and was not handicapped.

Martin was *handicapped*. A handicap is, by definition, a disadvantage for a given individual that limits or prevents the fulfillment of a normal role in life. Even with adjustments, accommodations and medication, he remained at a disadvantage and his life opportunities were sharply limited.

Developmental variations may be *disorders* or not. Variations may be problematic from time to time but they are not disorders because they aren't disabling or handicapping. Martin and Felix had disorders because they were disabled. What Henry and his father had were variations, not disabilities or disorders. They had problems with some stuff. So does everyone I have ever met.

Maybe that's just me and the company I keep, but I don't think so. I think it's the essence of the ADD problem. We use ADD to refer to variations, impairments, disabilities and handicaps. It is not only confusing, it robs the diagnosis of meaning.

I put all this in the note section because it's a bit turgid. It's a note to the personality chapter because developmental variations are the foundation of personality. Taking a broader perspective, developmental variations, personal strengths and weaknesses, are the cement that makes us who we are.

As we grow up, we learn to take advantage of our strengths and compensate for our weaknesses. Sometimes, our strengths are never even appreciated, let alone realized. Sometimes, we spend our lives contending with our weaknesses.

When you're old, you may realize that you'd have been wildly successful as a bond-trader or a crooner in the style of Michael Bublé. But no, you didn't know what your strengths really were and you followed your weaknesses. You wind up wasting your life as a second-rate psychiatrist. There was a lot of friction along the way. But, by what you deem the Grace of God, you wound up in a pretty good place. You found a lovely wife, you had six healthy children and your garden is full of flowers the year-round. We are, all of us, accumulations of differences and imperfections. No face is perfectly symmetric, no one has two identical hands, and no two snowflakes are the same. Differences and imperfections make us who we are, for better or worse.

It's the friction that arises along the way that we call disorders, although most often they are only transient problems, uncomfortable but not disabling. From time to time we experience anxiety or dismay, or your Central Executive goes off the rails for a bit.

I spoke of developmental variations, but in common language they are strengths and weaknesses, normal human differences and imperfections. They happen to be most apparent during development and maturation. They are amplified during that period because of an additional variable: the rate at which brain develops. They are also amplified during old age because the rate at which people decline also varies. In between, they are apparent during times of stress and struggle.

In developmental medicine we treat developmental variations that are disabling or handicapping. We also treat developmental variations that only cause mild problems, if only to relieve a child's transient suffering. We use terms like 'disorder', a term of convenience that is really quite vague and means a lot of things. It doesn't necessarily mean pathology. It only means that something isn't quite right. Every one of us is disordered in one way or another. Better not say, everybody has problems.

16, p25. *Nature has known about it for years.*

I didn't realize it myself until recently when I learned about something called *evolvability*. Humans are fast-evolvers. Our species is only 200,000 years old and look at how far we've come. We have digital watches, transistor radios and internal combustion engines. Not to mention vaccines, open heart surgery and the internet. Thus enthused, I dilated on the subject of evolvability in a scientific paper:

"Twentieth-century genetics was hard put to explain the irregular behavior of neuropsychiatric disorders. Autism and schizophrenia defy a principle of natural selection; they are highly heritable but associated with low reproductive success. Nevertheless, they persist. The genetic origins of such conditions are confounded by the problem of variable expression, that is, when a given genetic aberration can lead to any one of several distinct disorders. Also, autism and schizophrenia occur on a spectrum of severity, from mild and subclinical cases to the overt and disabling. Such irregularities reflect the problem of missing heritability; although hundreds of genes may be associated with autism or schizophrenia, together they account for only a small proportion of cases. Techniques for higher resolution, genomewide analysis have begun to illuminate the irregular and unpredictable behavior of the human genome. Thus, the origins of neuropsychiatric disorders in particular and complex disease in general have been illuminated. The human genome is characterized by a high degree of structural and behavioral variability: DNA content variation, epistasis, stochasticity in gene expression, and epigenetic changes. These elements have grown more complex as evolution scaled the phylogenetic tree. They are especially pertinent to brain development and function. Genomic variability is a window on the origins of complex disease, neuropsychiatric disorders, and neurodevelopmental disorders in particular. Genomic variability, as it happens, is also the fuel of evolvability. The genomic events that presided over the evolution of the primate and hominid lineages are over-represented in patients with autism and schizophrenia, as well as intellectual disability and epilepsy. That the special qualities of the human genome that drove evolution might, in some way, contribute to neuropsychiatric disorders is a matter of no little interest." (C. T. Gualtieri, 2021)

17, p26. *I wonder if ADDs make good hunters.*

Opposing views of hunters:

"Humans' survival depended on being (I) hypervigilant, including the ability to retrieve and integrate information through all senses at once-somewhat akin to parallel processing; (2) rapid-scanning; (3) quick to pounce (or flee); and (4) motorically 'hyperactive' (foraging for food, moving toward warmer climes as seasons and ice ages come and go, etc.), The 'response-ready' individual would likely have been advantaged under the brutal or harsh circumstances of the frozen steppe or humid jungle, whereas the excessively contemplative, more phlegmatic individual would have been 'environmentally challenged'."(Jensen et al., 1997)

"I questioned whether I would want to go hunting in a terrain that includes lions, venomous reptiles, and other potentially dangerous animals with someone who may be impulsive, disorganized, and accident-prone. I am not a hunter by trade, but from my limited education via National Geographic, it seems that hunting takes much patience, timing, and attention to details." (Triolo, 2001)

Jensen is talking about Henry. Triolo, about Martin.

Did you know that Neanderthals went extinct because they were ADD?

"We took advantage of the largest GWAS meta-analysis available for this disorder consisting of over 20,000 individuals diagnosed with ADHD and 35,000 controls, to assess the evolution of ADHD-associated alleles in European populations using archaic, ancient and modern human samples. Our analyses indicate that ADHD-associated alleles are enriched in loss of function intolerant genes, supporting the role of selective pressures in this early-onset phenotype. Furthermore, we observed that the frequency of variants associated with ADHD has steadily decreased since Paleolithic times, particularly in Paleolithic European populations compared to samples from the Neolithic Fertile Crescent. We demonstrate this trend cannot be explained by African admixture nor Neanderthal introgression, since introgressed Neanderthal alleles are enriched in ADHD risk variants. All analyses performed support the presence of long-standing selective pressures acting against ADHD-associated alleles until recent times. Overall, our results are compatible with the mismatch theory for ADHD but suggest a much older time frame for the evolution of ADHD-associated alleles compared to previous hypotheses." (Esteller-Cucala et al., 2020)

Although Hallowell and Ratey aver there is no evidence for an "attention deficit disorder (ADD) personality" and "ADD personality traits," they recognize the following abilities and attributes in individuals with ADHD: high energy, creativity, intuitiveness, resourcefulness, tenacity, hardworkingness (sic), a never-say-die approach, warm-heartedness, a trusting and forgiving attitude, sensitivity, the ability to take risks, flexibility, and a good sense of humor. (Hallowell & Ratey, 2013) Does that sound like a disorder?

18, p38. *Minds are built to wander freely.*

Neuroscientists have known for more than a century that the brain is active even when one is at rest; daydreamers have known it longer than that. When Hans Berger invented the electroencephalograph (EEG) in 1924, he noticed that the brain expressed electrical activity even when the subject was resting (alpha waves) or in deep sleep (delta). The brain was quiet but not silent; it never stopped. The importance of the discovery wasn't appreciated for a long time, except by the psychoanalysts, who always suspected that brain was up to something we didn't know about.

Critical studies of the state of relaxed mental awareness didn't begin until 50 years later, when David Lund, a Swedish physician, began to study regional blood flow in brain using radioactive isotopes; the precursor of PET and SPECT scanning. Studies of cortical blood flow patterns showed a hyper-frontal pattern in awake healthy subjects in the resting state, that is, high regional blood flow in the prefrontal cortex. He surmised the PFC was generating a state of conscious awareness. (Ingvar, 1979) It occurred, however, when the individual and his or her brain was in a resting state. Since it occurred when the individual wasn't doing anything but quietly resting, it was said to be the brain's default mode.

The idea that the brain might have a default mode, a state of activity when it isn't doing anything that engages its attention, struck many as absurd. When an organism isn't doing anything in particular, the activity of its brain is of no interest; or so it must have seemed to busy people who don't pay attention to things that just lie about not doing anything. Lying about in a state of idle reflection, however, is perhaps the most productive thing a brain can do. Think of Newton sitting under the apple tree, Descartes lying in bed or your brother-in-law in his ice-fishing hut. As one is just sitting there, his brain is not only active but is doing something. It is engaged in information processing. Without something to do, something that requires attention, we all have the experience of the mind wandering from one passing thought to the next. It seems like woolgathering, but it is meaningful, as we muse about past events and try to understand them, ponder what may happen in the future or imagine worlds that are far from our immediate surroundings. One is in brain's default mode; therein dwell fantasy, imagination, daydreams, and deep thought. (Raichle, 2010) (Buckner et al., 2008)

The brain's default mode occupies the default mode network. It is in the medial prefrontal cortex, the medial temporal lobe including the hippocampus, and parts of the cingulum and inferior parietal lobe; locations, as it happens, that are also components of the social/emotional brain.

The default mode elaborates experience. It is active during quiet moments when the only external information to process are leaves rustling in the trees or clouds floating by. Brain is not about to let such idle moments pass by staying idle itself. It capitalizes on them, consolidating past experience in ways that will prepare it for future events. Think of your laptop. You've turned off all your programs and it goes into sleep mode, but what it's really doing is thinking about itself. The little computer is looking after herself, backing up files, inserting patches into programs and updating her security. (Buckner et al., 2008)

Brain's default mode is events essential to oneself, and to others one is close to. It occupies itself like a pianist doing her scales, exercising an important function, reminding us who we are, where we stand with respect to others and why. It is scrapbooking, you could say, contemplating events in light of one's memories, sorting and arranging them according to their emotional valence, and trying to anticipate what might come of it all. The default mode almost always has someone else in there with you, or several others. Yet, curiously, it is also the seat of one's deepest thoughts and insights. Picture Socrates *standing all day in the market place lost in thought and oblivious of the external world*, with his head is in the clouds. (Buckner et al., 2008)

The default mode is not only a normal state but essential to health; apparently, we all ought to spend more time doing nothing. Patients whose default mode network is impaired are gravely disabled: patients with Alzheimer's disease and schizophrenia for example. (Broyd et al., 2009) Connections within the default mode network, particularly with the medial prefrontal cortex, are weak in patients with OCD, social anxiety and autism. (Hou et al., 2013) (Peterson et al., 2014) (Yerys et al., 2015)

In normal circumstances, the only way to modulate the activity of the default mode is to turn it off, and that happens automatically when one is involved in goal-directed activity. One wonders, then, if too much task-positive behavior can weaken one's default mode; or if a weak default mode network forces one to keep busy. In either event, a weak default mode undermines the foundations of who we are, what we do and why we do it. Socrates, his head not always in the clouds, said *Beware the barrenness of a busy life*.

19, p47. *Many other brain regions are also part of it.*

Damage to the frontal lobes (the prefrontal cortex in particular) leads to problems with concentration, perseverance, motivation, self-correction and impulse control, which also happen to be symptoms of ADD. That led us to suspect that ADD (MBD, as we called it in those days) was related to damage of dysfunction in the PFC. We wrote about this in a number of papers in the 1980s. (C. T. Gualtieri et al., 1983) (C. T. Gualtieri & Hicks, 1985) (R. W. Evans, Gualtieri, & Hicks, 1986) Subsequent studies have affirmed the theory. Other studies have pointed to brain abnormalities in other brain regions, such as the basal ganglia, cingulum and subcortical white matter. They only affirm the fact. Executive functions are usually said to reside in the prefrontal cortex, and they do, but like every neurocognitive function they involve a wider-ranging network that includes all those regions.

"The proposed model postulates a particular emphasis on the functional responsibilities of the frontal-striatal system. A neural substrate for the abnormal oscillations that characterize hyperactive children, the correction of which is germane to therapeutic stimulant effects, is presented in terms of the regulatory functions of the frontal lobe." (R. W. Evans, Gualtieri, & Hicks, 1986)

20, p48. *The prefrontal cortex is vulnerable to more than just trauma.*

The activity of the frontal cortex can be impaired by low oxygen at birth, by systemic diseases like chronic infections, high blood pressure, diabetes and auto-immune disease, by intense emotions, stress, overwork, sleep deprivation, idleness, alcohol and many other drugs, and by every mental illness.

An infant's brain is vulnerable to trauma and low oxygen supply around the time of birth. On an MRi, you can see tiny lesions in the deep white matter of brain. It happens because our brains are just too big for our own good. During the evolution of humans from the simian ancestor that we share with chimpanzees, the size of brain increased by a factor of three: from about 500 cc to around 1450. Unhappily, the brain's blood supply did not quite keep up. The white matter, in particular, is served by small arteries (arterioles) that take a tortuous course into the depths of brain. They are easily clogged. The white matter is a vast assembly of fiber bundles (axons) that connect nerve cells (neurons) from all over the brain. When the white matter is damaged, neurons don't develop quite so well as they ought to. The neurons of the prefrontal cortex are especially vulnerable to this kind of damage.

The reason why the PFC is so vulnerable is explained, indirectly, in Note 16. It's Darwinism.

21, p54. *Classifying normal childhood fears and worries as anxiety disorders.*

Mental illnesses are handicaps, a disadvantage that limits a person from living a normal life. They are severe conditions like intellectual disability, schizophrenia, Alzheimer's disease, OCD, manic-depression and some forms of depression. They are related to major problems in brain structure and function and tend to have a progressive, deteriorating course. They are comparatively uncommon but have occurred throughout history and in every culture.

Mental disorder is the term the DSM uses for every psychiatric condition. It doesn't make the crucial distinction between mental illness, mental disorders and mental problems. To me, a mental disorder is a disability, but not nearly so handicapping as chronic mental illness. It is a cognitive, emotional or behavioral disability that makes it difficult for a person to perform in the manner or within the range considered normal for a human being. ADD, anxiety and depression are mental disorders in some people, but not always. Sometimes they are handicapping, more often they are disabling but most of the timen they're just problems.

Addictions begin as problems, then become disabling (disorders) and then handicapping (chronic mental illness).

Mental problems are what we all have from time to time, small but sometimes troublesome impairments in cognition, emotion or behavior. They are usually transient and people usually get better on their own, like many cases of ADD.

The mental problems that bring patients to consult a specialist have always changed from one generation to the next, and they vary in different cultures. Our understanding of what is a mental disorder has also varied over time and place. Mental illnesses, on the other hand, are constant across times and cultures.

The DSM uses 'mental disorder' to cover every psychiatric

condition, and for its own very good reasons. What is necessary for psychiatric research, epidemiologic surveys and insurance filings, however, is often confusing to the laity.

Children are prone to mental illness, but not very often. The most severe childhood conditions are congenital, originating before birth, such as the Fragile X syndrome and other neurogenetic syndromes. They are associated with intellectual disability and the most challenging extremes of behavior and emotion. Schizophrenia may occur in pre-pubertal children, but not very often. Childhood bipolar disorder is a myth. The mental illnesses that afflict adults, like schizophrenia, manic-depression and OCD usually begin during adolescence or early adult life. (Jones, 2013)

Children are prone to mental disorders, because that is what the DSM calls them. In the DSM, a disorder is "A clinically significant behavioral or psychological syndrome or pattern that occurs in an individual (that) is associated with present distress (e.g., a painful symptom) or disability (i.e., impairment in one or more important areas of functioning) or with a significantly increased risk of suffering death, pain, disability, or an important loss of freedom." The definition does not distinguish mental disorders from mental problems like inattention, which are less severe and less persistent, or from mental illness, like schizophrenia, which is chronic and disabling. The word 'distress' necessarily imparts subjectivity to the diagnostic process.

During early development, behavior and emotional problems abound. For that reason, research usually indicates higher rates of mental disorders in children compared to adults, including depression, anxiety, suicidal thoughts and OCD. The disparate rates prove the point; most of the behavior and emotional problems of childhood abate or dissipate after puberty. Children who are anxious do not necessarily grow up to be anxious adults, and children who are unhappy don't always become depressed adults. Autistic children tend to be less autistic during adolescence. The childhood disorder with the highest rate of continuity into adult life is conduct disorder – children who are antisocial and aggressive. But only half of conduct disorder children grow up to be antisocial adults. There is an essential discontinuity between the psychological problems of children and those of adults.

There are plenty of continuities between childhood and adult life, enough to satisfy the researchers who want to find them. People who develop mental illnesses in adult life often have had mental problems during childhood, like anxiety, an awkward manner, temperamental behavior and hyperactivity, but the relationships are weak and non-specific. One can't predict that a child with such problems will grow up and be mentally ill or, if so, what mental disorder will occur. Several generations of psychiatric research have assiduously sought the childhood precursors of mental illness and with small success.

Nevertheless, the continuity of childhood and adult disorders has been a prevailing theme in psychiatry since the study of children began in earnest, at the turn of the last century – *As the twig is bent, so grows the oak*. But people aren't oak trees and, besides, there are many other things that influence the growth of oak trees besides just bending the twig.

Years ago, a prominent child psychiatrist wrote: "Neurotic disorders in children (unhappiness misery, anxiety, fears, obsessions, and the like) can be distressing and handicapping. If at all severe or persistent, neuroses undoubtedly warrant treatment. However, perhaps surprisingly, child neurosis is not usually a precursor of adult neurosis. Indeed, it may be that to some extent they constitute different sorts of disorder in spite of rather similar symptomatology. The prognosis for most neuroses in childhood is very good. The great majority of neurotic children become normal adults and, contrary what one might expect, the risk of manic-depressive disorder or anxiety neurosis in adult life appears to be no different in neurotic children from that in the general population. At present, little is known on how to distinguish the small minority of child neuroses that become chronic." (Rutter, 1970) Nothing has changed since then.

22, p55. *An anxious person finds it hard to maintain his attention to a specific task.*

"Anxiety reduces available central executive capacity. The most important distinction in processing efficiency theory is between effectiveness and efficiency. Effectiveness refers to the quality of task performance indexed by standard behavioral measures (generally, response accuracy). In contrast, efficiency refers to the relationship between the effectiveness of performance and the effort or resources spent in task performance, with efficiency decreasing as more resources are invested to attain a given performance level. Negative effects of anxiety are predicted to be significantly greater on processing efficiency than on performance effectiveness.

"When an individual perceives him- or herself to be under threat and so experiences anxiety, it is potentially dangerous to maintain very high attentional control to a specific stimulus or location. Instead, the optimal strategy is to allocate attentional resources widely, thereby reducing attentional control with respect to any ongoing task. Of central importance to the revised theory is the notion that anxiety decreases the influence of the goal-directed attentional system and increases the influence of the stimulus-driven attentional system

"According to attentional control theory, the adverse effects of anxiety on the inhibition function mean that anxious individuals are more distracted than nonanxious ones by external task-irrelevant stimuli presented by the experimenter and by internal task-irrelevant stimuli (e.g., worrying thoughts; self-preoccupation)." (M. W. Eysenck et al., 2007)

23, p55. *The most trivial stimulus will seize their attention.*

"From a clinical perspective, cognitive theories of anxiety have emphasised the role of biases in attentional processes in the aetiology and maintenance of anxiety states... Anxiety is characterised by a hypervigilant mode in which the person scans the environment for threat-related stimuli, with priority of processing being allocated to the initial encoding of threat. Individuals differ in their readiness to adopt a vigilant processing mode for threat, with those vulnerable to anxiety having a greater tendency to direct processing resources towards danger-relevant stimuli.

"High trait anxious individuals tend to react to increased activation of threat input units by switching resources towards the source of threat, whereas low trait anxious individuals have a bias to direct processing resources away from an item that has been evaluated as threatening. Thus, the direction of the attentional bias for threat provides an index of vulnerability to generalised anxiety." (Mogg et al., 2000)

"An important approach to treatment that relates the neural circuits of attention to anxiety disorders is attention bias modification therapy. The central notion of this therapy is that anxiety and its disorders result in part from the failure of the orienting network to disengage from stimuli related to anxiety. Pathologies of anxiety may emerge either through overactivity in the emotion affect networks or from the inability to disengage from negative ideas because of problems in attention networks." (Ghassemzadeh et al., 2019)

24, p55. *More difficulty generating energy in their prefrontal cortex.*

"Anxious individuals show deficits across a range of non-affective tasks that place demands on attentional or cognitive control. The data reported here suggest that trait anxiety is associated with deficient recruitment of DLPFC mechanisms that are used to augment attentional control in response to processing conflict... This impoverished recruitment of prefrontal attentional control mechanisms was observed using a purely cognitive task in the absence of threat related stimuli. It should also be noted that this deficient recruitment was primarily associated with trait and not state anxiety, suggesting that it reflects a processing style or deficit that is associated with vulnerability to anxiety rather than a symptomatic outcome of altered mood state.

"At a broad level of analysis, the account put forward here shares certain commonalities with attention control theory in suggesting that anxious individuals are characterized by deficient attentional control, particularly when inhibition of distractor processing is required. Contrary to ACT, however, we propose that this deficit is associated with reduced, rather than increased, DLPFC recruitment." (S. Bishop et al., 2004) (S. J. Bishop, 2009)

25, p56. *Stress hormones impair the activity of mitochondria.*

"The brain has the highest energy consumption (around 20% of our body oxygen and 25% of our glucose) while just representing 3% of our body's mass... Biological conditions which involve subtle mitochondrial alterations would have a negative impact on brain functions, increasing vulnerability to brain disorders... Individuals with suboptimal mitochondrial function would be particularly vulnerable to stress-associated depletion of the brain's energy resources and, hence, to the development of psychopathologies. The stress hormones glucocorticoids are produced and metabolized by mitochondria and, conversely, mitochondrial function is affected by glucocorticoids and other metabolic stress mediators. Accordingly, mitochondrial functioning would be intimately linked to mechanisms of stress adaptation and regulation...Highly anxious states may affect mitochondrial function through the actions of glucocorticoids and other metabolic stress mediators." (Filiou & Sandi, 2019)

"Glucocorticoids play an important biphasic role in modulating neural plasticity; low doses enhance neural plasticity and spatial memory behavior, whereas chronic, higher doses produce inhibition... After 3 days of treatment, high, but not low, doses of CORT resulted in decreased GR and Bcl-2 levels in mitochondria. As with the in vitro studies, Bcl-2 levels in the mitochondria of the prefrontal cortex were significantly decreased, along with GR levels, after long-term treatment with high-dose CORT in vivo." (Du et al., 2009)

26, p57. *How to explain that anxiety sometimes responds to stimulant drugs?*

1. As per (23) and (25), there are reasons to believe that attentional mechanisms are not quite right in anxiety patients.

2. Stimulants improve the efficiency of the Central Executive. One is less likely to be distracted by worrisome extraneous events.

3. Anxiety saps one's mental energy. Stimulants increase it.

4. When one is fatigued or mentally drained by anxiety, stimulants have an alerting effect and convey a sense of well-being.

5. There are so many kinds of anxiety and so many ways people turn into worriers, there is no therapy or drug that doesn't help some of them.

27, p59. *Milo had writer's block, right?*

We don't know very much about writer's block. Writing is a complicated endeavor but that isn't the only reason why most people hate to write. An old theory is that writing is putting oneself to paper, an act that makes one vulnerable. Oddly, people don't seem to have the same qualms about exposing a whole lot more of themselves on social media. Writing is hard work, it is tedious and ranks only next to lectures as something to get distracted from. Creative writing – inventing characters and a story – is particularly challenging; we don't always have a story to tell and some writers never do. There are people who like to write and to them a bad case of writer's block must be hellish. Some people are hypergraphic, meaning that they write all the time. They are typically patients with manic-depression or an interesting kind of epilepsy. I can't imagine what writer's block would be like in someone with hypergraphia.

28, p60. *The counsellor suggested it might be ADD.*

Milo didn't have ADD, of course. Mental blocks are sometimes diagnosed as stress reactions and they are sometimes linked to stress but not always. They are usually dissociative reactions (aka conversion disorder or hysteria). A patient with conversion disorder wakes up to discover he can't move his legs; there is no neurological reason why he can't but his mind won't let him. Writer's block occurs in accomplished writers. She is certainly able to put pen to paper, as they used to say, but something in her mind won't let her. The expanse of brain that generates writing has been dissociated or blocked from the part of brain that says, *Do it*. OCs in general and perfectionists in particular are prone to dissociative reactions.

29, p63. *At the level of elementary neurobiology.*

ADD and OC are both identified with the prefrontal cortex but also reside in the basal ganglia, thalamus and the cingulum. In ADD, the network is not active enough. In OC, it is too active.

For example, the cingulum.   The front part of the cingulum is involved with error detection and performance monitoring and also the regulation of attention and emotion. OCs have an over-active cingulum but ADD patients have a cingulum that is less active in performance monitoring and error processing. The cingulum is the major white matter pathway connecting to the cingulate cortex, whose anterior portion is an area which has been repeatedly implicated as abnormal in ADD, in terms of smaller volumes, slower rate of thinning in adolescence, decreased activity on task-based functional MRI, and decreased functional connectivity. The cingulum has been found to have diffusion abnormalities in ADHD adults. (Cooper et al., 2015)

29, p64. *I wrote about ADD adults in 1985.*

"Twenty-two adults who met DSM-III criteria for Attention Deficit Disorder, Residual Type (ADD-RT) were evaluated in a series of clinical experiments. Although certain personality and psychological factors typified the ADD-RT group, methylphenidate blood levels, the growth hormone response to methylphenidate, and the brainstem evoked response did not distinguish subjects from matched controls. Male subjects seemed to be a more homogeneous group than female subjects. Socioeconomic status and IQ, but not severity of ADD symptoms, were found to predict outcome. ADD adults seem to be numerous and easy to identify, at least on the basis of symptoms. However, the validity of ADD-RT as a 'distinct clinical entity' is open to question." (C. T. Gualtieri et al., 1985)

30, p68. *The central executive is weak from the very start and remains so.*

Patients with ADD have persistent deficits during adult life, but they are not the same as they were when they were kids. They learn to compensate for and sometimes overcome their early deficits. A study that we did in a large group of relatively bright and advantaged ADD patients, children, adolescents and young adults, indicated that even successful compensation comes at a price.

We examined how the cognitive abilities of ADD patients changed with age, compared to normal adults. In normal people, every test improved with age. ADD patients, however, demonstrated a different pattern. Their performance improved with age in tests of psychomotor speed (FTT and SDC) and sustained attention (CPT), but not in important components of the two tests of executive control, the Stroop test and the shifting attention test.

On the Stroop test, reaction times grew faster with age in normal individuals but not in ADD patients. In both groups, the number of errors decreased with increasing age. Normal controls were able to improve their performance, however, and also to increase the speed with which they responded. ADD patients were no faster at age 29, however, than they were at age 10.

This pattern was demonstrated more dramatically on the shifting attention test, a more rigorous test of cognitive flexibility. In both groups, the number of correct responses improved with age, and so did the error rate. However, normal individuals achieved better scores with faster reaction times, and the correlation between reaction time and age was negative. ADD patients, however, were able to better their performance as they matured, but only by adopting a comparatively inefficient strategy. Their response times were slower; they were less efficient.

"Our data support cognitive inefficiency as an important element in the ADD syndrome. In absolute terms, the difference between adult ADD's and adult normals on the SAT was 142 msecs. One hundred and forty-two msecs is not a very long time. In a car driving 60 MPH, it is only 12.5 feet. Activating a response on your PC by pressing a key takes 17 msecs. In the life of a neuron, though, it is a long time.

"In the life of an individual, what is the cumulative impact of a 142 msec increment in every complex mental operation he or she undertakes? What is the bio-energetic cost? What is the opportunity cost? And how is that reflected in the psychology of a person? The cumulative effect of slower information processing speed probably represents a significant burden to the ADD adult. An organism so heavily taxed might be prone not only to cognitive difficulties, but behavioral and emotional complications as well." (C. Gualtieri & Johnson, 2006)

31, p69. *The numbers are higher than during three previous, unlamented amphetamine epidemics.*

There have been occasions in the past when amphetamines were prescribed liberally by physicians, comparable to what American physicians have been doing for the past 20 years: in Sweden in the 1940s and the US in the 60s. The only difference is that, in those days, amphetamine wasn't prescribed for ADD or cognitive enhancement, but for weight loss, depression and anxiety, pain and fatigue. Most of the patients were women.

Prior to 1971, amphetamines were prescribed freely and physicians' offices had free samples to distribute. A national survey conducted that year found that amphetamines were used by 6.5% of American adults.   Among the ten million Americans who used amphetamines in 1970, 40% used them 'non-medically', that is, obtained without a prescription, and 20% were said to 'abuse' the drugs. Almost a million (10%) met 'some criteria of dependence' and 320,000 were said to be addicted – 3.2% of all users.

In 1938, amphetamine was introduced in Sweden, and a year later it required a prescription. In 1942, approximately 3% of the Swedish population had a prescription for amphetamine, while the vast majority used under five amphetamine tablets per year, about 3,000 citizens were known to take it daily and among them about 200 used over 10 amphetamine tablets per day. In 1942, amphetamine was added to the list of controlled substances. Gradually the supervisory authority, the Royal Medical Board, made more stringent recommendations for prescribing narcotic drugs.

At the end of World War II in 1945, Japanese drug companies were left with hundreds of thousands of pounds of military-made liquid methamphetamine left over from the war. They mounted advertising campaigns to encourage consumers to purchase the over-the-counter medicine. Sold under the name "wake-a-mine", the product was pitched as offering "enhanced vitality". With an estimated 5 per cent of Japanese between the ages of 18 and 25 taking the drug, many became intravenous addicts. There were at least 200,000 amphetamine addicts in Japan by 1954. (Rasmussen, 2008)

32, p73. *Taking methylphenidate or amphetamine may have adverse effects on a pregnancy.*

Stimulants are among the most commonly used prescription medications in pregnancy. In 2015, 1% of pregnant women were taking prescribed stimulants, mostly for ADD. (Louik et al., 2015) The number is probably higher now. Women planning to become pregnant are routinely advised to discontinue medications that they don't really need, but it seems that a lot of women feel they need ADD meds.

Are stimulants safe to use during pregnancy? Maybe or probably – I can't say for sure. A definite answer isn't available. The Food and Drug Administration classifies ADHD medications in "pregnancy category C"; that means there is "insufficient information to confirm either harm or lack of harm."

What we know about stimulants in pregnancy is mostly from studies that were done during the crack cocaine epidemic. In the late 1980s and early 1990s, an estimated 100,000 babies exposed to cocaine were born in the United States *every year*. In some urban, low-SES areas, as many as 18 percent of live births were 'crack babies'. (Minnes et al., 2011) There was deep concern at the time. At birth, babies whose mother used crack cocaine were smaller and more irritable. They were likelier to have been born prematurely. (Ladhani et al., 2011) As infants, they were found to have subtle neurological abnormalities. Years later, they were still a bit smaller; they also had small but significant behavioral and neurocognitive problems. (Wouldes et al., 2004)

Prenatal cocaine exposure does not have teratogenic effects and severe disabilities do not result; that much is re-assuring.

With respect to the impact of minor deficits, we simply don't know. Isolating the effects of cocaine on development and maturation is virtually impossible, in light of the many baleful influences of households where one or both parents use cocaine and in neighborhoods where crime and drug use is rife. The same problems obscure the effects of maternal methamphetamine use. Meth babies show the same pattern of growth effects and subtle neurological deficits as crack babies but the children grow up in environments that are similarly disadvantaged. (Good et al., 2010) The methodological problems are formidable: how to attribute bad outcomes to (1) cocaine and meth or, (2) the genes of drug-abusing parents or (3) the effects of growing up in dubious circumstances.

Nevertheless, human children are resilient and early growth retardation and mild neurological deficits can be overcome in a good-enough if not optimal environment. A lingering question, however, is posed by the 'Developmental Origins of Health and Disease' theory. (Barker, 1995) A large body of research suggests that a suboptimal uterine environment is associated with the occurrence of adult disease, most notably cardiovascular disease and perhaps also dementia. (Whalley et al., 2006) (Muller et al., 2016) Low birth weight, for example, is associated with adult health and smaller brain volume seven decades later. (Wheater et al., 2020) The statistical associations are by no means predictive, but whether or not the theory is entirely correct, pregnant women are wisely encouraged to take extraordinary steps – avoiding processed meats, caffeine, DEET and most drugs – in order to provide the developing fetus an optimal uterine environment.

The experience of babies exposed to cocaine or methamphetamine may not be relevant to pregnant women who continue to take methylphenidate or amphetamine for ADD. They take much lower doses of stimulants that are less potent and less toxic than cocaine and methamphetamine. Further, if high daily doses of the most toxic stimulants have only small effects, doesn't that suggest that low doses of methylphenidate or amphetamine are safe to take during pregnancy?

There have been studies of ADD meds and their fetal effects, but the results are not decisive. There are reports that the babies of mothers who take stimulants for ADD are likelier to be born preterm, are smaller (Huybrechts et al., 2018), have lower APGAR scores (Bro et al., 2015) and are more likely to be treated in the neonatal ICU. (Nörby et al., 2017) The rate of fetal loss both may be increased with methylphenidate. (Besag, 2014) The risks are very small, however, and the findings are complicated by the fact of maternal ADD itself; "Because women who were treated with ADHD drugs before or after pregnancy also clearly differed from nonusers, the underlying disease or lifestyle aspects might be important factors that are difficult to control for." (Nörby et al., 2017) Many adults treated with stimulants for supposed ADD have other or additional mental disorders.

Stimulants in pregnancy are not associated with congenital malformations, even among crack or methamphetamine mothers; for a long time, the same was said to be true for ADD mothers on methylphenidate or amphetamine. (Dideriksen et al., 2013) (Besag, 2014) (Nörby et al., 2017). More recently, however, there have been reports of "a small increase in the risk of cardiac malformations associated with intrauterine exposure to methylphenidate but not to amphetamines" (Huybrechts et al., 2018); of malformations in general with methylphenidate (Kolding et al., 2021); and of malformations with methylphenidate and amphetamine. (Anderson et al., 2020)

"Meta- analysis of 4 cohort studies with almost 3000 women exposed to methylphenidate only, and almost 3 million unexposed controls, yielded an OR of 1.26 (95 % confidence interval 1.05-1.51) for major malformations, and 1.59 (95 % confidence interval 1.02-2.49) for cardiac malformations. In conclusion, methylphenidate exposure in early pregnancy is associated with a small but significant increased risk for major malformations, which can be attributed mostly to increased risk of cardiac malformations." (Koren et al., 2020)

The rates are very small, but statistically significant. The recent data were generated by studies of entire populations whose medical data was culled from electronic databases. The data are compelling until one appreciates that information in databases is not comprehensive and may not include other salient data, like maternal diagnosis, concomitant use of alcohol or illicit drug use. Even when large databases were analyzed, very few of the mothers used stimulant drugs; the small numbers compromised the validity of the results. (Nörby et al., 2017) (Anderson et al., 2020)

It is odd that malformations may occur with ADD meds taken in low doses but have not been observed in the babies of cocaine and methamphetamine users. I have no idea why methylphenidate is more likely to be associated with malformations than amphetamine; the pharmacology of the drugs is not notably different. In experimental animals, cocaine and methamphetamine are clearly fetotoxic, but methylphenidate isn't, even at very high doses. (Teo et al., 2003) One concludes that the risk of fetal malformation is very low if it occurs at all.

BTW, the amounts of methylphenidate secreted in breast milk and consumed by the infant are very small but the same may not be true for amphetamine. (Ornoy, 2018).

Are stimulants for ADD safe to use during pregnancy? One answers with a negative: one cannot assume that they are safe but evidence that they are unsafe is marginal. The appropriate question is, Do you really *need* to take them?

33, 73. *Women who use marijuana during pregnancy.*

Cannabis is the most frequent illicit substance consumed by pregnant women. World estimates range from 3 to 30% of pregnant women.(Metz & Stickrath, 2015) In 2013, the US rate was 3.4% of pregnant women and in 2017 it was 7%. (Volkow et al., 2019) It is probably higher now, and the potency of cannabis preparations is higher than ever. Contemporary marijuana products have higher quantities of delta-9-tetrahydrocannabinol than in the 1980s when much of the marijuana research was completed.(Metz & Stickrath, 2015)

Twenty-one states of approve the use of legal cannabis for nausea and vomiting including its use in pregnancy. (O'Connor, 2018)

Marijuana freely crosses the placenta and is found in breast milk. Despite the widespread use of cannabis by young women, there is limited information available about the impact perinatal cannabis use on the developing fetus and child, particularly the effects of cannabis use while breast feeding. (Jaques et al., 2014) However, data are far from uniform regarding adverse perinatal outcomes. Existing studies are plagued by confounding by tobacco and other drug exposures as well as sociodemographic factors. (O'Connor, 2018) "Women who used marijuana were younger; more likely to be of African American race; had inadequate prenatal care; and use tobacco, alcohol, and other drugs. After adjusting for smoking, other drug use, and African American race, the composite and all individual markers of poor neonatal outcome were not significantly higher among women who used marijuana during pregnancy." (Conner et al., 2015)

Cannabis may have adverse effects on both perinatal outcomes and fetal neurodevelopment. Specifically, marijuana may be associated with fetal growth restriction, stillbirth, preterm birth, and NICU treatment after birth. (El Marroun et al., 2009) (Hayatbakhsh et al., 2012) (Warshak et al., 2015) (Gunn et al., 2016)

"Cannabis does not act as a classical teratogen and is not associated with morphological abnormalities at birth. Fetal exposure has been associated with changes in physical growth and maturation early in life but long-term growth, including pubertal milestones, are unaffected. Global intelligence scores in children with a history of in utero cannabis exposure are typically not affected but aspects of cognition involved with executive functioning (e.g. attention, inhibitory control, planning) can be negatively impacted. Effects of exposure also include higher levels of depression and anxiety during adolescence, suggesting that psychological outcomes may be particularly sensitive to the disrupting influence of gestational cannabis exposure. Results from preclinical modeling studies have confirmed that in other mammalian species, fetal exposure to THC does not result in changes in long-term physical growth but may negatively impact certain aspects of cognition, and heighten the occurrence of behaviors that are consistent with anxiety. While the neurodevelopmental effects of in utero cannabis exposure are subtle, they are persistent and have been observed in more than one species. Pregnant women should not assume that it is safe to use cannabis during pregnancy." (Grant et al., 2018)

34, P74. *We don't share cannabis with little babies.*

"Ganja tea is one of many 'bush teas' that comprise the inventory of household medicines and remedies in rural Jamaica where mothers care for their families with a repertory of home-based and folk practices. Prepared and served in the privacy of the home, even middle-class families occasionally consume ganja in this form. In fact, men who have acquired social status often shift their form of consumption from smoking to tea drinking without seeming to experience any conflict. And women who adamantly warn their husbands and sons about the dangers of ganja smoking nevertheless prepare ganja infusions routinely for their entire households, including the youngest of children.

"Although there is a variety of opinion about the optimal age for initiating children to ganja tea, ranging from birth to toddler age, all women agreed that the teas must be titrated carefully in accordance with the child's age and previous experience with ganja. Thus, younger children first receive a weak version of the tea, perhaps only a leaf steeped in hot water, after which the child is observed and the strength of the tea adjusted accordingly. Gradually the strength is increased to reach adult levels of potency sometime in early adolescence. When asked about the possibility of making the tea too strong, mothers reported that this occasionally does happen and is evidenced by two somewhat opposite reactions on the part of their children: sleepiness and hyperactivity.

"The most commonly mentioned child health problems for which ganja infusions are used are colds. Other childhood health problems that informants claimed could be ameliorated by ganja included infant diarrhea, marasmus, anorexia, colic, asthma, bronchial wheezing, croup, the discomfort of teething, and hyperactivity. Several caretakers had at least one story of how ganja had solved a problem, relieved discomfort, or saved a life without the benefit of a physician or when physicians were unable to help.

"Another reason given for preparing ganja tea for children is to enhance the learning potential of children. According to the homemakers interviewed, ganja does this by increasing their power to concentrate on schoolwork, to pay attention to what the teacher is saying, not to be distracted by schoolmates or the activities of other classes, to remain quiet and serious in class, to carry out homework assignments even when very tired, and to sit for examinations. Ganja often is referred to as the Wisdom Weed that, according to legend, was discovered growing on King Solomon's grave. In contrast, teachers who were interviewed were much more guarded in their opinions about ganja. They gave examples of children who had been good students but whom ganja had made 'lazy,' 'careless,' or even 'mad' or 'criminal.' Most of the teachers said that they had 'heard' that ganja tea was helpful in times of sickness but uniformly rejected the notion that ganja would improve school performance." (Dreher, 1984)

35, P78. *I've never known anyone to die from ADD.*

Apparently, some people think it happens. This dubious statistic is often referenced: "ADHD-drivers have an almost fourfold risk of (motor vehicle) accident compared to non-ADHD-drivers". (Barkley et al., 1993) (Cox et al., 2006) Subsequent studies have lowered the odds from 4 to 1, then to 2 to 1 and then 1.2 to 1. (Redelmeier et al., 2010) (Liu et al., 2021) So, instead of 400% more likely to have a crash, their risk is only 20% higher. The increased risk is likely explained by the fact that people with ADD happen to drive more. Those who actually do have accidents usually have additional problems, like epilepsy, antisocial behavior and substance abuse. (Vaa, 2014) (Liu et al., 2021)

"The assertion that ADD-drivers violate traffic laws more often than other drivers should be modified: ADD-drivers do have more speeding violations, but no more drunk or reckless driving citations than drivers without ADD. All accident studies included in the meta-analysis fail to acknowledge the distinction between deliberate violations and driving errors. The former are known to be associated with accidents; the latter are not. A hypothesis that ADHD-drivers speed more frequently than controls because it stimulates attention and reaction time is suggested." (Vaa, 2014)

People with ADD are slightly more death prone than non-ADDs. The old data has them almost twice as likely to die in accidents, by homicide or by suicide. (Klein et al., 2012) (Barbaresi et al., 2013) (Dalsgaard et al., 2015) (London & Landes, 2016) The most recent information makes them 7% more likely. (Chen et al., 2019) It comes from Taiwan, where the prevalence of ADD is 1.2%, considerably lower than in the US. (Wang et al., 2016) One assumes more conservative diagnosing in Taiwan and that most of the ADDs there are severe cases (i.e., MBDs).

No study has reported increased death rates from natural causes. Among the garden-variety USA-brand of ADDs, there is no mortal danger to the disease, untreated. If a bad accident occurs, it is more likely to be an ADD patient who has additional, more severe problems.

36, P80. *Punding*

Not many words have made their way from Swedish to English -- think *Ombudsman* and *Smorgasbord*. Punding is another. It is slang for 'blockhead'. It refers to what amphetamine and cocaine addicts do. They have an intense fascination with common objects, which are repetitively manipulated, examined, collected, sorted, and stored. Like emptying one's purse, sorting and cleaning the contents, putting them all back in order, then doing it again and again. It occurs most often these days in patients with Parkinson's disease who take dopaminergic drugs like L-DOPA and in patients with dementia.

37, P82. *Addiction*

The word has become too harsh for the sensitive ears of 21st century citizens. So, we have *substance abuse*, a general term that simply describes injudicious use of a substance. A *substance use disorder* is a DSM-5 term that lumps addiction with other forms of hazardous drug use. *Misuse* is a term commonly met with in medical papers. It means that a drug is used without a prescription, without medical supervision and for a non-medical purpose. A college student who borrows his friend's Adderall to prepare for exams is, by definition, misusing the drug. But he is using much less than Elspeth and Karl, both of whom got Adderall from a physician.

38, p85. *Less than 61% of the managers.*

"No fewer than 61% of the managers said they cancelled social engagements because of information overload." (Waddington, 1996)

"The people who don't are said to be better at 'prioritizing and winnowing'." (Berner, 2007)

39, p92. *Stimulant drugs enhance cognitive flexibility or the ability to multitask.*

Studies have shown that ADD children improve on measures of cognitive flexibility when they take a stimulant. It is an indirect effect. Patients with ADD have problems with attention, memory and processing speed, and stimulants go a long way towards correcting those deficits. As a result, they will do better on just about any cognitive test you can give them, including IQ tests and the SATs. Patients like Marcia and Rebecca aren't ADD. Their minor problems on the CNT were well within the range of normal. When they took a stimulant, they experienced the non-specific effects of the drug: alertness, increased energy, relief from fatigue and a sense of well-being.

40, p106. *Stimulating effects attributed to their effects on dopamine and norepinephrine.*

"Stimulants increase extracellular levels of norepinephrine, dopamine, and to varying degree, serotonin. Importantly, the qualitative and quantitative neurochemical actions of these drugs are dependent on both the identity and dose of drug. For example, cocaine potently affects serotonergic neurotransmission, whereas amphetamine increases extracellular serotonin levels only at moderately high doses and methylphenidate has minimal impact on serotonin across a broad range of doses. Combined, these observations indicate that enhanced serotonergic neurotransmission is not an essential mechanism underlying the arousal-enhancing actions of psychostimulants, although this may contribute to the arousal-enhancing actions of certain stimulants.

"Microdialysis studies demonstrate a close relationship between amphetamine-induced waking/arousal and amphetamine-induced increases in norepinephrine and dopamine efflux. Additionally, it is now clear that both norepinephrine and dopamine exert robust wake-promoting actions. The wake-promoting effects of norepinephrine involve synergistic actions of alpha1- and beta-receptors, whereas dopamine-induced waking involves both D1 and D2 receptors. Finally, additional studies have identified subcortical regions involved in the wake-promoting actions of both norepinephrine and amphetamine. These regions include, but may not be limited to, the medial septal area, the medial preoptic area, and the lateral hypothalamus. Combined, these and other observations indicate a prominent involvement of both norepinephrine and dopamine in stimulant-induced arousal via actions within a network of subcortical regions."(Berridge, 2006)

"Dopamine and norepinephrine systems do not represent separate compartments within the CNS but rather an interconnected system, which share key neurobiological features making it as the endogenous circuitry where amphetamines electively impinge to produce a number of systemic effects. The strong anatomical connections between NE and DA systems are conserved at molecular level. This is best represented by the phylogeny of NE and DA transporters, which represent the evolutionary divergence of an archaic single catecholamine transporter (meNET), which was isolated and characterized in the brain of the teleost fish, Medaka." (Ferrucci et al., 2019)

41, p108. *CART is neuroprotective.*

"CART (cocaine- and amphetamine-regulated transcript) peptides (CART 55-102 and CART 62-102) are peptidergic neurotransmitters that are widely but specifically distributed throughout the brain, gut and other parts of the body. They are found in many brain regions associated with drug addiction including the nucleus accumbens, ventral tegmental area and ventral pallidum. Injections of CART 55-102 into the nucleus accumbens have no effect on basal locomotor activity. However, an injection of CART just before an i.p. injection of cocaine reduces the locomotor activating effects of cocaine. These and other data suggest that CART in the accumbens blunts the effects of cocaine. A hypothesis is that CART is homeostatic in the accumbens and tends to oppose large increases in dopamine signaling. These actions would therefore be able to regulate the effects of some abused drugs such as the psychostimulants." (Hubert et al., 2008)

42, p110. *TBI patients are treated with stimulants but not wisely.*

The commonest mistakes are to use stimulants too early in the course of brain injury recovery, when they have little effect; and to use doses that are too low to have an effect (e.g., 5 or 10 mg of Ritalin or Dexedrine – most TBI patients are young adults, and need higher doses). Stimulants are often given to patients who have had concussions – mild brain injuries. Concussion patients rarely need any medication at all. We will only treat concussion patients if they are still symptomatic 4, 5 or 6 months after the injury.

43, p114 *The research is dubious.*

"Neuroimaging studies show structural alterations in several brain regions in children and adults with attention-deficit/hyperactivity disorder (ADHD). Through the formation of the worldwide ENIGMA ADHD Working Group, we addressed weaknesses of prior imaging studies and meta-analyses in sample size and methodological heterogeneity. Our sample comprised 1713 participants with ADHD and 1529 controls from 23 sites (age range: 4-63 years; 66% males). Individual sites analyzed magnetic resonance imaging brain scans with harmonized protocols. Case-control differences in subcortical structures and intracranial volume (ICV) were assessed through mega- and meta-analysis. The volumes of the accumbens (Cohen's d=-0·15), amygdala (d=-0·19), caudate (d=-0·11), hippocampus (d=-0·11), putamen (d=-0·14), and ICV (d=-0·10) were found to be smaller in cases relative to controls. Effect sizes were highest in children, case-control differences were not present in adults. Explorative lifespan modeling suggested a delay of maturation and a delay of degeneration. Psychostimulant medication use or presence of comorbid psychiatric disorders did not influence results, nor did symptom scores correlate with brain volume. Using the largest data set to date, we extend the brain maturation delay theory for ADHD to include subcortical structures and refute medication effects on brain volume suggested by earlier meta-analyses." (Hoogman et al., 2017)

44, p116. *Normal brain is subject to mini-strokes.*

The small arteries deep in the brain tend to get clogged even in the best of us. You usually don't experience them as TIAs or mini-strokes but they are apparent on an MRi: 'White matter hyperintensities, normal for age.' Well, they may be normal (as in normative) because everyone has a few, but most of us would prefer a less ischemic side of normal.

45, p119. *Caffeine drinkers are less likely to develop dementia.*

"With a history that began in 800 A.D., coffee is the most popular drink known and as a result, the issues regarding its physiologic effects deserve attention. Maintaining alertness is a well-known benefit and in addition, the cardiovascular (CV) effects of the active compounds, which include polyphenols and caffeine, must be considered. Genetics are relevant and where slow caffeine metabolism is inherent, the risk of nonfatal myocardial (MI) has been shown to be increased. Overall risk for coronary heart disease (CHD) is not supported and unless there is excessive intake, congestive heart failure (CHF) is not adversely affected; in moderation, there may be some benefit for CHF. There is no apparent increased risk of sudden cardiac death (SCD). Overall, there also appears to be a beneficial inverse association with all-cause mortality, although this is not absolute for extra heavy intake. Benefit in reducing stroke also has supportive evidence. Hypertension is not increased by coffee. Boiled and unfiltered coffee appears to increase plasma cholesterol and triglycerides but for the overall metabolic syndrome, there appears to be benefit. There is also some evidence that paper-filtered coffee results in an increase in some markers of inflammation. Association of coffee with arrhythmias has been a major concern though in moderation it is not a significant overall problem. Therefore, only if a patient were to associate major arrhythmic symptoms with coffee would cessation have to be advised. Where coffee clearly shines from a CV standpoint is in the established decrease in onset of type 2 diabetes mellitus (DM). Any benefit or harm has always been attributed to caffeine as the apparent major component. However, coffee contains a myriad of compounds, including polyphenols. These other substances may be most relevant for potential benefit or harm and some of these may be partially removed or altered by coffee preparation methods such as paper filtration. Multiple studies support this by what appears to be no CV advantage or disadvantage for decaffeinated coffee. The bottom line on coffee, for those who enjoy the brew, is that it is a wonderful beverage with rare associated CV disadvantage and with much to recommend it from an overall CV standpoint." (Eskelinen & Kivipelto, 2010)

"Caffeine has well-known short-term stimulating effects on central nervous system, but the long-term impacts on cognition have been less clear. Dementia and Alzheimer's disease (AD) are rapidly increasing public health problems in ageing populations and at the moment curative treatment is lacking. Thus, the putative protective effects of caffeine against dementia/AD are of great interest. Here, we discuss findings from the longitudinal epidemiological studies about caffeine/coffee/tea and dementia/AD/cognitive functioning with a special emphasis on our recent results from the Cardiovascular Risk Factors, Aging and Dementia (CAIDE) study. The findings of the previous studies are somewhat inconsistent, but most studies (3 out of 5) support coffee's favorable effects against cognitive decline, dementia or AD. In addition, two studies had combined coffee and tea drinking and indicated some positive effects on cognitive functioning. For tea drinking, protective effects against cognitive decline/dementia are still less evident. In the CAIDE study, coffee drinking of 3-5 cups per day at midlife was associated with a decreased risk of dementia/AD by about 65% at late life. In conclusion, coffee drinking may be associated with a decreased risk of dementia/AD. This may be mediated by caffeine and/or other mechanisms like antioxidant capacity and increased insulin sensitivity. This finding might open possibilities for prevention or postponing the onset of dementia/AD." (Eskelinen & Kivipelto, 2010)

"Moderate coffee consumption was inversely significantly associated with CVD risk, with the lowest CVD risk at 3 to 5 cups per day, and heavy coffee consumption was not associated with elevated CVD risk." (Ding et al., 2014)

"Epidemiologic studies indicate that coffee consumption reduces the risk of Parkinson's disease and Alzheimer's disease. To determine the factors involved, we examined the protective effects of coffee components. We found that quercetin, flavones, chlorogenic acid, and caffeine protected SH-SY5Y cells from these toxins. They also reduced the release of tumor necrosis factor-α and interleukin-6 from the activated microglia and astrocytes and attenuated the activation of proteins from P38 mitogen-activated protein kinase (MAPK) and nuclear factor kappa light chain enhancer of activated B cells (NFκB). After exposure to toxin containing glial-stimulated conditioned medium, we also found that quercetin reduced oxidative/nitrative damage to DNA, as well as to the lipids and proteins of SH-SY5Y cells. There was a resultant increase in [GSH]i in SH-SY5Y cells. The data indicate that quercetin is the major neuroprotective component in coffee against Parkinson's disease and Alzheimer's disease." (Lee et al., 2016)

"To evaluate the associations between coffee and caffeine consumption and various health outcomes, we performed an umbrella review of the evidence from meta-analyses of observational studies and randomized controlled trials (RCTs). Of the 59 unique outcomes examined in the selected 112 meta-analyses of observational studies, coffee was associated with a probable decreased risk of breast, colorectal, colon, endometrial, and prostate cancers; cardiovascular disease and mortality; Parkinson's disease; and type-2 diabetes. Of the 14 unique outcomes examined in the 20 selected meta-analyses of observational studies, caffeine was associated with a probable decreased risk of Parkinson's disease and type-2 diabetes and an increased risk of pregnancy loss. Of the 12 unique acute outcomes examined in the selected 9 meta-analyses of RCTs, coffee was associated with a rise in serum lipids, but this result was affected by significant heterogeneity, and caffeine was associated with a rise in blood pressure. Given the spectrum of conditions studied and the robustness of many of the results, these findings indicate that coffee can be part of a healthful diet." (Grosso et al., 2017)

46, p120. *Useful for treating late life depression and early dementia.*

"The most frequent use was the combination of methylphenidate with citalopram in four trials for depression, showing significant improvement of the patients' symptoms, as assessed by the Hamilton Depression Rating Scale], and good tolerability. Other eleven trials were conducted for different conditions: post-stroke depression, Parkinson's disease, falls age-related cognitive decline, post-stroke rehabilitation, and medically ill patients with depressive symptoms.

"Regarding the studies focused on patients with dementia, all participants had clinical improvement. Four studies described trials aiming to evaluate the efficacy of methylphenidate in the treatment of apathy in patients with Alzheimer's disease; one study evaluated the efficacy of methylphenidate in the treatment of hypothermia in patients with dementia with Lewy's bodies; one case study assessed the efficacy of methylphenidate in the treatment of frontotemporal dementia and finally, one trial assessed the efficacy of methylphenidate in patients with dementia and negative symptoms which included reduced interest in self-care, work and home tasks, social and family interaction." (Sassi et al., 2020)

47, p121. *Older people are at particular risk for heart attack.*

"A study of patients 65 years of age and older who were taking ADHD medications showed increased risk of 1 case of new heart failure per 10.5 person-years of stimulant use, with the symptoms usually appearing within the first 90 days of initiation of the ADHD medication. Not surprisingly, older patients were far more likely to present with new heart failure or cardiomyopathy than younger patients, and the older patients tended to present earlier after ADHD drug initiation. ADHD medications have been associated with acute coronary syndrome in the setting of normal coronary arteries on angiography. Stress-induced cardiomyopathy, also referred to as Takotsubo cardiomyopathy, has also been reported in patients taking ADHD medications." (Torres-Acosta et al., 2020)

47, p124. *Theoretically, that would increase the efficacy or side effects of both.*

A 3 mg dose of cannabis combined with 10 mg of amphetamine increases the subjective high but also increases blood pressure. (M. A. Evans et al., 1976) (Petersen, 1980)   Cannabis and amphetamine have a pharmacokinetic interaction; amphetamine is metabolized by the liver under the action of the enzyme, CYP2D6. CYP2D6 is inhibited by THC, CBD and CBN, with CBD being the most potent. (Alsherbiny & Li, 2019)

Most stimulant interactions are pharmacodynamic. Stimulants are sympathomimetic drugs. That means they mimic the actions of the sympathetic nervous system. Such drugs increase heart rate, blood pressure and cardiac output (epinephrine, midodrine, dopamine); dilate the bronchial tree (albuterol); dry the nasal mucosa (phenylephrine, ephedrine, pseudoephedrine, terbutaline); and diminish appetite (phentermine, phenmetrazine). Taking a stimulant with another sympathomimetic drug increases the risk of side effects, especially heart attack and stroke. Phenylpropanolamine was a popular decongestant that was banned because of side effects, including acute hypertension and hemorrhagic stroke. However, ephedrine and pseudoephedrine also increase the risk of stroke, and so can sprays that contain phenoxazoline or oxymetazoline. (Cantu et al., 2003) Strokes have also occurred in users of supplements containing ephedra alkaloids (e.g., ma huang). Any supplement advertised as a memory-booster, energizer, weight-reducer or life-extender may well contain a sympathomimetic chemical, and you won't know it.

In 2020, a survey of more than 9 million US adults reported that 3% had been prescribed stimulants and about half of them were taking at least one additional psychoactive drug and a fourth were using two or more. Extrapolating to 300,000,00 American adults, 9,000,000 were taking prescription stimulants and more than 4 million were on one or more additional psychoactive drug. 48% were taking antidepressants, 31% were taking sedatives and 20% were taking opioids. (T. J. Moore et al., 2023)

Stimulants also interact with most antidepressants, sometimes enhancing their effects and sometimes increasing side effects. Some antidepressants are more sympathomimetic than others – bupropion, desipramine, venlafaxine, duloxetine and all the monoamine oxidase inhibitors. (Markowitz & Patrick, 2005)

Taking a stimulant and a sedative drug is dubious practice. *Uppers in the morning and a downer at night.* Stimulants enhance the analgesic and euphoric effects of opioids and decrease opioid-induced sedation. They do the same with alcohol.

48, p125. *Maybe it will kill you.*

"We conducted a retrospective analysis of the Nationwide Inpatient Sample data (2010–2014). Patients (aged 15–22 years) with a primary diagnosis for acute myocardial infarction (AMI) (N = 1,694) were compared with non-AMI (N = 9,465,255) inpatients for odds ratio (OR) of substance use by logistic regression model, adjusted for demographics, medical risk factors, and comorbid substance use.

"Tobacco (28.4%) and cannabis (14.9%) use were most prevalent in AMI inpatients. Cocaine (OR = 3.9), amphetamine (OR = 2.3), and cannabis (OR = 1.3) users were at higher risk of AMI hospitalizations. Higher proportion of cannabis users (14.7%) had major severity of illness at admission and higher mean total charge compared with that seen in cocaine and amphetamine users. Angioplasty was used more in cannabis users (19.4%) than others. The in-hospital mortalities were 2.7% and 2% in overall AMI cohort and cannabis users, respectively, and none in cocaine and amphetamine users." (Patel et al., 2020)

"This is a register-based cohort study of 20,581 individuals in treatment for illicit substance use disorders in Denmark between 1996 and 2006. All in all, 1441 deaths were recorded during 111,445 person-years of follow-up. Standardized mortality ratios (SMRs) for primary users of specific substances were: cannabis: 4.9, cocaine: 6.4, amphetamine: 6.0, heroin: 9.1 (CI: 8.5-9.8), and other opioids 7.7 (CI: 6.6-8.9)." (Arendt et al., 2011)

When cannabis and amphetamine are administered together to

lab rats, cannabis actually *protects* the rats from amphetamine addiction. I can't imagine what an amphetamine-addicted rat is like, but it doesn't sound good. However, in human substance abusers (aka addicts) cannabis + amphetamine increases the likelihood of brain damage, cognitive impairment and psychosis. Cannabis might be good for your addicted pet rat, but high doses of cannabis + amphetamine are demonstrably dangerous.

"Animal studies showed mostly protective effects of both CBD and THC upon amphetamine exposure in models used to investigate several phases of amphetamine addiction (e.g. drug-seeking, relapse, extinction), and neurobiological markers (e.g. neurotoxicity, brain damage)... Overall, for amphetamine-induced mental health, there was a CBD-related protective effect for amphetamine-induced animal models of psychosis. Also, CBD and THC protected against amphetamine-induced brain damage.

"In contrast, studies in human mostly showed counter-protective effects or no effect on the co-use of cannabis with amphetamine for several outcomes, including brain (e.g. MRS, MRI), mental health, cognition (e.g. neuropsychological performance, psychotic symptoms) and amphetamine use. Overall, brain structure and metabolism studies showed that cannabinoids co-use with methamphetamines is associated with neurotoxicity and abnormal brain function." (Daldegan-Bueno et al., 2022)

49, p127. *40% of such patients were impaired on at least one of our cognitive tests.*

"Patients with anxiety, depression, and bipolar disorder are known to be impaired relative to healthy controls on neurocognitive tests, but the degree of impairment may be obscured if the data are analyzed in terms of group means. Patients and controls were administered a comprehensive neurocognitive assessment that measured performance in 5 domains: memory, psychomotor speed, reaction time, attention, and cognitive flexibility. Clinic patients diagnosed per DSM-IV-TR criteria with generalized anxiety disorder (N = 63), major depressive disorder (N = 285), and bipolar I or II disorder (N = 96) were compared with 907 controls. Subjects' age range was 18 to 65 years. Patients had no comorbid psychiatric disorders and no medical, neurologic, or developmental conditions that might affect cognition (e.g., attention-deficit/hyperactivity disorder, brain injury, mild cognitive impairment, chronic pain). Data on patients and controls (collected from March 2003 through February 2007) were taken from a clinical database that also contained neurocognitive test scores. There were small differences between patients and controls, between different patient groups, and between treated and untreated patients when neurocognitive results were compared in terms of group means. Comparisons of results in terms of the frequency with which patients and controls fell below certain cutoff scores amplified the importance of these differences. Only 4% of controls fell below a standard score of 70 (2 standard deviations below the mean) on 2 or more cognitive domains, but 19% of anxiety patients, 21% of depressed patients, and 30% of bipolar patients fell below the standard score. Substantial numbers of patients with anxiety, depression, and bipolar disorder are cognitively impaired. A score that is 2 standard deviations below the mean is usually clinically important, and 2 domain scores in that range is cause for serious concern. The importance of this finding is discussed, with respect to clinical trials, in terms of establishing a homogeneous trial population and minimizing the placebo response rate." (C. Gualtieri & Morgan, 2008)

51, p130. *Perhaps I will share it with you someday.*

OK, OK. If you must know...

Take a large number of smart, energetic kids who want to devote their lives to fighting disease and alleviating suffering. Make them spend four years of the usual college debauch in their dorm rooms sweating for a 3.9 GPA. That cuts the number of potential physicans down by three-fourths. Then subject them to 7-14 additional years of study and training that are even more oppressive. Along the way, give them examinations that are fiendishly difficult. Some require months (sic) of preparation. Then, as they can finally celebrate the fruits of their labors, subject them to periodic re-examinations, audits and 'peer reviews' by physicians who should have read my OC book. Not to mention the patient satisfaction surveys. (*That doctor dint refill my Adderall. Ahm dis-satisfied.*)

Did anyone tell those kids that that fighting disease and alleviating human misery would entail working for venture capitalists or large, voracious hospital corporations? Or that the silicon-paperwork burden is enervating? Or that one is required to run patients through the clinic as if they were cattle?

We are oppressed!

Also, if you read my OC book, you'd know that some OCs are oppressed by their perfectionistic natures. And just about every physician is a bit OC.

51, p134. *Psychosis as a possible stimulant side effect.*

Not too long ago, a study reported that psychosis occurred in 2.4 of every 1000 patients age 13 to 25. Amphetamine was a more likely culprit, compared to Ritalin. (Moran et al., 2019) The study was published in an influential medical journal. It failed to acknowledge that the median point and 12-month prevalence of psychosis in that age group is 3.89 and 4.03 per 1000 persons respectively and the median lifetime prevalence is 7.49 per 1000 persons. (Moreno-Küstner et al., 2018) Does it mean that stimulants *reduce* the risk of psychosis?

52, p136. *Their activity is under exquisite control.*

"Beginning with the genomic DNA, evidence exists for the

transcriptional regulation of tyrosine hydroxylase mRNA levels, alternative RNA processing, and the regulation of RNA stability. There is also experimental support for the role of both translational control and enzyme stability in establishing steady-state levels of active tyrosine hydroxylase protein. Finally, mechanisms have been proposed for feedback inhibition of the enzyme by catecholamine products, allosteric modulation of enzyme activity, and phosphorylation-dependent activation of the enzyme by various different kinase systems. Given the growing literature suggesting that different tissues regulate tyrosine hydroxylase mRNA levels and activity in different ways, regulatory mechanisms provide not only redundancy but also diversity in the control of catecholamine biosynthesis." (Kumer & Vrana, 1996)

53, p137. *Stimulants are not good for depressed patients who may be suicidal.*

"By specific drug class, the adjusted models suggest lifetime nonmedical use of prescription pain relievers, stimulants, and depressants for males were significantly related to suicidal ideation, but not suicide attempts for pain relievers and stimulants. For females, the adjusted models also suggest lifetime nonmedical use of prescription pain relievers, stimulants, and depressants were significantly related to suicidal ideation, but not suicide attempts for pain relievers. However, both nonmedical use of stimulants and depressants were significantly related to suicide attempts." (Zullig et al., 2015)

"149 studies were eligible and 59 were included in meta-analyses. There was significant heterogeneity in effects. Evidence came mostly from cross-sectional studies. Any use of amphetamines was associated with higher odds of psychosis (odds ratio [OR] $=2.0$), violence (OR $=2.2$), suicidality (OR $=4.4$) and depression (OR $=1.6$). Having an amphetamine use disorder was associated with higher odds of psychosis (OR□=□3.0),violence (OR□=□6.2),and suicidality (OR□=□2.3).(McKetin et al., 2019)

54, p139. *Reports of 25 sudden deaths in people taking stimulants.*

"Although the committee recognized that there are important potential benefits of these drugs for certain highly dysfunctional children, we rejected the notion that the administration of potent sympathomimetic agents (i.e., amphetamines) to millions of Americans is appropriate. We sought to emphasize more selective and restricted use, while increasing awareness of potential hazards. ADHD medications should be prescribed only after safer options, such as regular exercise and omega-3, have been considered and/or tried." (Nissen, 2006)

"The US Food and Drug Administration (FDA) collected 25 anecdotal reports of sudden death documented during industry-sponsored medication trials as well as those reported for individual patients to the FDA. The mechanism that led to the sudden death of these patients is unknown. "The frequency of sudden unexpected death among those taking stimulants is no higher than that in the general population of children. Only 19 children and adolescents of the 2.5 million taking stimulants died suddenly over 5 years, suggesting a base rate among children and adolescents of 4 incidents of sudden death per year per 2.5 million children or fewer than 2 incidents per million; however, reported rates of SCD in the general child and adolescent population are substantially higher, with reports varying from 8 to 62 per million." (Perrin et al., 2008)

"Even modest increases in BP and HR have been associated with increased risk of adverse cardiovascular events. In the meta-analysis carried out by Mick et al. on 2665 adult patients, it was observed that CNS stimulants used for adult ADHD were associated with a statistically significant increase in resting heart rate of 5.7 bpm and increase in systolic blood pressure of 1.2 mmHg but not of diastolic blood pressure. A low overall risk

(≤5%) of clinically significant cardiovascular events, including tachycardia or hypertension, was also observed. Epidemiological studies have demonstrated that elevated resting heart rate is a significant independent predictor of mortality and a shorter life expectancy. Cooney et al. demonstrated that 15 bpm increase in heart rate was found to increase the rate of cardiovascular disease mortality by 23–50% in men and women. Perret-Guillaume et al. showed that heart rate increase of 10 bpm is associated with a 20% increased risk of cardiac death. HR increases comparable with those observed with CNS stimulant treatment for adult ADHD have been associated with a 17% increased cardiovascular mortality and about 8% in those with coronary artery disease. In another study carried out by Wilens et al., statistically significant change in systolic blood pressure by about 5 mm Hg and diastolic blood pressure of about 7 mm Hg was observed. Blood pressure variations of this magnitude, in particular during long-term therapy, have been acknowledged to increase morbidity and mortality." (Sinha et al., 2016)

55, p139. *No reason to believe that routine EKG screening prevents sudden death.*

"Children, adolescents, or adults who are being considered for treatment with stimulant medications should have a careful history (including assessment for a family history of sudden death or ventricular arrhythmia) and physical exam to assess for the presence of cardiac disease and should receive further cardiac evaluation if findings suggest such disease (e.g., electrocardiogram and echocardiogram). Patients who develop symptoms such as exertional chest pain, unexplained syncope, or other symptoms suggestive of cardiac disease during stimulant treatment should undergo a prompt cardiac evaluation." (The package insert for all psychostimulant drugs.)

"The American Academy of Pediatrics recommends a careful assessment of all children, including those starting stimulants, by using a targeted cardiac history (e.g., patient history of previously detected cardiac disease, palpitations, syncope, or seizures; a family history of sudden death in children or young adults; hypertrophic cardiomyopathy; long QT syndrome) and a physical examination, including a careful cardiac examination.

"Given current evidence, the AAP encourages primary care and subspecialty physicians to continue currently recommended treatment for ADHD, including stimulant medications, without obtaining routine ECGs or routine subspecialty cardiology evaluations for most children before starting therapy with these medications." (Perrin et al., 2008)

"Hypertrophic cardiomyopathy (HCM) is the most common cause of SCD in the United States in people 30 years old or younger. The disease prevalence has been estimated as high as 1 per 500 in young adults. It is typically non-obstructive and presents in mid to late adolescence. HCM is often clinically silent, but the ECG typically may show left ventricular hypertrophy or T-wave abnormalities. The diagnosis traditionally has been best confirmed by echocardiography. Associated sudden death is often exertional and is usually secondary to malignant ventricular arrhythmias... Restriction from most competitive athletics is recommended in patients with HCM.

"Cardiovascular screening for conditions that could lead to an increased risk of sudden death has focused mainly on the pre-participation screening of athletes. In the United States, current recommendations are for a focused personal and family history of the athlete with special emphasis on history of exertional chest pain, syncope or a family history of early sudden death, as well as examination for blood pressure, murmurs, and stigmata of Marfan's syndrome. If any abnormalities are found, additional studies are initiated to systematically exclude known causes of sudden death. A relatively intense debate has been ensuing over the effectiveness of universal electrocardiogram (ECG) screening for athletes and/or all infants. For the past 25 years in Italy, all athletes have undergone ECG) screening, with some data indicating fewer deaths during athletic activities associated with institution of the screening program. Although the reduction in SCD has been related to disqualification of young people found to have HCM, ARVC and other rare abnormalities, the current reported rate of SCD (about 0.8/100,000 per year) is not very different from that reported for unscreened athletes in the United States. These data and the relatively large number of estimated eligible athletes in the United States that would require screening (10-12 million) have led to the current recommendations against universal ECG screening in the US. The cost of the ECG and its interpretation, in addition to further testing due to frequent false positive results, has been determined to have an unfavorable cost-benefit ratio." (Gajewski & Saul, 2010)

56, p141. *Amphetamine can precipitate or aggravate atrial fibrillation.*

"As the population ages globally, atrial fibrillation (AF) is predicted to affect 6–12 million people in the USA by 2050 and 17.9 million in Europe by 2060. The reasons for the increase in the prevalence of AF remain elusive and are related to multiple factors including: enhanced detection, increased incidence, and greater survival after onset of AF." (Morillo et al., 2017)

"At age 55 and older, the lifetime risk of atrial fibrillation is about one in five; this risk rose to more than one in three in individuals with at least one of the following risk factors: cigarette smoking, alcohol misuse, hypertension, obesity, diabetes, myocardial infarction, and heart failure." (Staerk et al., 2018)

"Abnormal sympathetic and parasympathetic cardiac inputs secondary to stimulant use can result in increased myocardial excitability and conductance. Patients with exaggerated sympathetic nervous system activity are more susceptible to develop clinically significant cardiac arrhythmias typically more in the setting of an underlying structural heart defect. There are very few reports associating amphetamine-dextroamphetamine therapy to new onset atrial fibrillation and atrial flutter." (Sinha et al., 2016)

57, p142. *Stimulants are not innocuous in adults.*

"Both stimulant and nonstimulant catecholaminergic medications used in adults with ADHD are associated with minor, but statistically significant, changes in heart rate and blood pressure that were often observed in those receiving placebo. Given the minor pressor and chronotropic effect of these medications, adults with ADHD should have their blood pressure and heart rate checked at baseline and periodically during treatment." (Wilens et al., 2005)

"Seven of the ten studies included in this systematic review did not find an association between prescription stimulant use and adverse cardiovascular outcomes. Six of the seven studies of children and adolescents did not find an association between prescription stimulant use and adverse cardiovascular outcomes. Low incidence of adverse cardiovascular outcomes among children and adolescents in the general population hampered these studies. In adults, however, a safety signal—prescription stimulant use associated with adverse cardiovascular outcomes—was demonstrated in two of three studies. More suggestive of a safety signal, studies of adults found an increased risk for transient ischemic attack and sudden death/ventricular arrhythmia." (Westover & Halm, 2012)

"Using the Sentinel distributed database, we analyzed new-onset heart failure or cardiomyopathy among initiators of selected ADHD medications (amphetamine products including lisdexamfetamine, methylphenidate, and atomoxetine). The highest rates occurred soon after treatment initiation in the age group 65 years or older, with 1 case per 10.5 person-years of follow-up, or 950 cases per 10,000 person-years, for days 0–90." (Mosholder et al., 2018)

"We conducted a retrospective matched cohort study to assess the odds of a cardiovascular event among individuals with ADHD exposed to amphetamine compared with individuals with ADHD who were not exposed to this medication. During the index period of January 1, 2018, through December 31, 2020, 13,233 individuals older than 65 years (mean age = 69 years) met the study criteria.

"The cohort exposed to amphetamine had increased blood pressure and increased odds of cardiovascular events (odds ratio [OR], 6.16; absolute risk difference = 3.31%) compared with the control group.

"Amphetamines have clear safety data in younger age cohorts; however, this safety data may not generalize to older populations. Additional research is warranted to clarify further exposure and subpopulation-level risk factors associated with adverse cardiovascular events among older patients." (Latronica et al., 2021)

58, p143. *Legislative action to channel cognitive-enhancement technologies.*

We need laws to allow mentally competent adults to use as much Ritalin, Adderall, Dexedrine modafinil, centrophenoxine, piracetam and ginkgo biloba as they want. Why didn't I think of that? (Maher, 2008) (Greely et al., 2008)

59, p144. *College students have little difficulty getting a stimulant prescription.*

College students don't have to get prescriptions, either. They get stimulants easily enough from friends or family. (McCabe & Boyd, 2005) The non-medical stimulant use rate – kids who take stimulants they obtain without a prescription -- is 5-10% in American high schools and 5-35% in colleges. (McCabe et al., 2004) (McCabe et al., 2006) (Wilens et al., 2008) (Clemow & Walker, 2014) (Smith & Farah, 2011) A 2005 survey found that

26% of college students with prescriptions for methylphenidate had given or sold some of their medication at least once (Teter et al., 2006) and two more recent surveys reported that 60% of college students with stimulant prescriptions shared stimulants with peers. (Garnier et al., 2010) (Gallucci et al., 2015) Researchers have done wastewater analyses on college campuses; someone has to do the dirty work. Metabolites of amphetamine and methylphenidate increase by 760% (!) during finals week of the second semester. (Burgard et al., 2013) (D. R. Moore et al., 2014)

"Overall, 18 % (198/1,115) of this medical student sample had used prescription psychostimulants at least once in their lifetime, with first use most often in college. Of these, 11% (117/1,115) of students reported use during medical school (range 7–16 % among schools)." (Emanuel et al., 2013) Other surveys have put the rate as high as 50%.

CHAPTER 25. WHAT STIMULANTS DO

60, p148. *Everyone knows what attention is.*

Attention is the solution to the problem of a limited input space. Conscious awareness has limited processing capacity; it is a processing bottleneck. At a point in time, only so much noise can be transmuted into signal; an effective mind has to assign priorities to incoming stimuli. This is the function of attention; it converts sensation into perception. By definition, it is a regulatory function that governs the interface between sensation and perception. It is a filter that attenuates extraneous mental operations and maintains others in awareness. Attention operates at the interface between awareness and all the other cognitive functions including memory, processing and motor control.

"Attention is a relatively broad cognitive concept that includes a set of mechanisms that determine how particular sensory input, perceptual objects, trains of thought, or courses of action are selected for further processing from an array of concurrent possible stimuli, objects, thoughts and actions. Selection can occur in a top-down fashion, based on an item's relevance to the goals and intentions of the observer, or in a bottom-up fashion, whereby particularly salient stimuli can drive shifts of attention without voluntary control." (Talsma et al., 2010)

61, p154. *Mental processing speed is how fast the brain can think.*

Reaction time is a way to measure mental speed:

This is a simple reaction time task: *Press the button as soon as you see the light go on.* The train of events is this: 1, sensation: the light comes on and you see it; 2, perception: you recognize the sensation as a light; 3, analysis: you remember the instruction and decide what to do; and 4, motor response; you press the button. Not a hard test, you have to agree. It's not hard to recognize a light or remember an instruction you were just given. It's *simple* reaction time, after all. But it's not so simple inside your head and there are several things brain must do to get it done. Also, it's not instantaneous. A 30-year-old human at the peak of his or her cognitive powers, takes about 285 milliseconds to get the job done. In contrast, the blink of an eye is 25 milliseconds. A healthy 80-year-old takes 381 milliliseconds because reaction times get slower with age. Also, individuals vary in mental speed. Runella's simple reaction time was as slow as an 80-year-old's. When we test elite athletes, we are not surprised to see simple reaction times as fast as 150 milliseconds.

Now, make the test more complicated. This is complex reaction time: *Press the button as soon as you see a red light on the screen, but don't press for a light of any other color.* Steps 1 and 4 are exactly the same, seeing the light and pressing the button. Step 2, perception requires an additional step – *What color is the light?* Step 3, analysis, entails a decision – *Do I press the button for this light, or not?* It's not hard, but it takes a healthy 30-year-old brain no less than 575 milliseconds to get around to pressing the button, and an 80 year-old, 710 milliseconds. An additional 290-329 milliseconds are needed to make simple color discrimination and a binary decision. During that additional time, about 300 milliseconds, brain is processing information and deciding how to act on it. In other words, it is *thinking*. The speed of thought, or mental processing speed, in this choice reaction time test, is 300 milliseconds. It is the speed of *central processing* or just plain processing speed.

What is happening during those 300 milliseconds? A signal is traversing the length of neurons in the form of an electrical current. At the synapse, the junction between one neuron and the next, the transmission is chemical. The presynaptic neuron releases a neurotransmitter, a small molecule that activates the post-synaptic neuron.[*] That takes one or two milliseconds. When the post-synaptic neuron is activated (an action potential), it takes about 14 milliseconds for the signal to travel its entire length, from its receiving end (the dendrite), across the cell body and then down its sending unit, the axon. Does that mean that during the 300 milliseconds needed for perceptual discrimination and decision-making, the signal must traverse 19 neurons?

If only it were so simple. Neurons don't behave as if they were chained together. On the receiving end, neurons have five or so dendrites, each of which has innumerable branches. It is said to be a 'dendritic tree' because its branches stretch out in every direction. The neuron is receiving signals from thousands of other neurons. At the other end, the axon *arborizes*, forming branches and twigs that make contact with about 10,000 other neurons.[†]

---

[*] A synapse is where one neuron touches another. Neurotransmitters are released from the presynaptic neuron and activate the post-synaptic neuron, whereupon they are sucked up by the presynaptic neuron (reuptake) and recycled.
[†] An action potential spreads along the axon of the presynaptic neuron; the axon arborizes and its branches form synapses with thousands of postsynaptic neurons.

Even in a simple cognitive exercise – *red light > press the button* -- untold millions of neurons participate in the event. Yet the signal gets through, as if it were travelling in a straight line. It happens because neurons know what to do. They respond only to some signals. Begin with the neurons that recognize the signal. They fire in response to the red light, but not just once. They fire a succession of action potentials successively, and at specific frequency. The signal is carried by neurons firing in a specific pattern. The firing pattern can be considered a code for red light, but it is really a wave. The properties of the wave, its waveform, is what carries information. The waveform is only recognized by neurons that can contribute to the exercise. Most neurons fail to recognize the waveform and decline to participate, which is OK because they have nothing to offer. The waveform carrying the signal, red light, ultimately meets the waveform that is one's memory of the instruction. The waves intersect and generate a new waveform, the signal that prepares motor neurons to press the button.

What is happening is the formation of an *ad hoc* neural network. It's not a chain, but a network of neurons, most of which are contributing to the exercise in indirect ways. Some neurons in the network maintain your level of alertness and motivation during the task. Some are monitoring your performance to make sure you do right. Other neurons contribute small changes to the waveform that may make it go faster or operate more efficiently. Still others suppress unwanted perceptions like *What a stupid test this is* or the sounds your stomach is making or the sounds the graduate student is making, the guy who is giving you the test, as his stomach is growling.

A lot is going on during those 300 milliseconds, you must admit. A host of neurons are activated and others are bypassed. A neural network forms to carry relevant information and does so as an electrical wave front.[‡] Your experience of this stupid test

---

[‡] We can actually measure the properties of the wave front with a

it is a two-step process -- *Aha. Red light. Press the button.* In fact, your experience is a brain field of inordinate complexity.

The speed with which all this happens is fast in some people and slow in others. It depends on anatomical factors. These differ among individuals and they also account for individual differences. Neurons are coated with an insulating substance called myelin, and thick myelin makes electrical signals course more rapidly along dendrites and axons. Children don't have fully-formed myelin sheaths around their neurons, which is why their reaction times are slower. Patients with multiple sclerosis lose the myelin coating around their neurons; slow reaction times are the earliest cognitive signs of MS. Neurons with more spines on their dendrites and axons are faster and more efficient, and thick spines are faster than thin ones. Intelligent people have thicker spines. Neurons with more synapses work faster; old people have fewer spines and synapses and patients with dementia lose spines and synapses at an astonishing rate.

The speed and efficiency of mental processing speed is also influenced by chemical factors, and here our friends, dopamine and norepinephrine, play a key role. They are ordinarily described as neurotransmitters; the molecules that make neuronal connections in the synapse. They are, but only in small, circumscribed regions of brain. Their more important role is *neuromodulators*, and in this role they regulate the activity of large brain areas. Dopamine and norepinephrine float in the watery fluid that surrounds nerve cells. Floating about, they find receptors in the axons and dendrites of neurons – receptors that are not in the synapse. Once they bind to one of those receptors, they set in motion a number of changes within the neuron itself, affecting the way proteins and ions behave and even influencing the expression of neuronal DNA. They do so on the scale of seconds or minutes. But once

---

technique known as Evoked Potentials; the technique is used when one has to test sight and hearing in infants who may be blind or deaf.

those changes are made within the neuron, neuronal speed and accuracy increases.

The take-home message is that amphetamines enhance neuronal communication and speed it up, probably because they stimulate dopamine. Its slow action as a neuromodulator allows more than enough time to allow neuronal networks to form and to generate a wave front of synchronized neurons. The wave front of thousands of neurons is the neural basis of perception, decision-making and action. In one experiment, dopamine increased the speed of this process from 300 to 100 milliseconds.

62, p159. *What they learned, they remembered.*

"Fourteen children with Attention Deficit Disorder with Hyperactivity (ADD + H) were administered the psychostimulant methylphenidate in a double-blind, placebo-controlled, crossover study. Subjects were evaluated on a well-validated measure of verbal memory and learning with an experimental design comprised of four conditions: placebo and active drug at three doses. Positive memory effects were found in the drug conditions. Significant dose-response relationships were found, indicating enhanced learning from placebo to low to medium to high dose. However, there was a differential drug effect on the memory task; methylphenidate selectively enhanced storage and retrieval mechanisms without affecting immediate acquisition." (R. W. Evans, Gualtieri, & Amara, 1986)

63, p160. *There is nothing to consolidate.*

Something is deemed worthy to remember. That may or not be a deliberate process. Some memories are formed at random. The first stage in memory is *encoding*; a brain signal is formed and exists in a labile, transient form. The signal resides, we think, in the hippocampus, a small brain region that is degraded in early Alzheimer's disease. The signal is easily erased by subsequent memories. *Henry, let me introduce you. This is Bob, and Mary, Dick, Jane and Runella.* You encode each of those names, but each new one erases the memory of the one before. The only name you remember is Runella.

The Runella signal in your hippocampus is consolidated but not Bob, and Mary, Dick or Jane. That means the signal moves from the hippocampus to create a memory trace in a network of neurons. Memory consolidation involves, among other things, the generation of proteins in the network, but we don't know how stimulants improve memory storage. It has something to do with norepinephrine, maybe.

"Modulatory influences on consolidation include release of norepinephrine (NE) within the amygdala. For example, foot-shock stimulation induces NE release in the amygdala; administration of epinephrine or drugs that enhance consolidation increases NE release in the amygdala; and the use of drugs that impair decreases NE release. Most important, amphetamine infused into the amygdala after training enhances memory of both types of training." (McGaugh, 2000)

Once memory is consolidated, it is harder to erase although it may degrade and disappear over time. Unless you rehearse the memory: *Runella. Runella. Where have I heard that name before?*

64, p164. *They don't have positive effects on memory, etc.*

"The effect of dopamine on the activity of prefrontal neurons is complicated, involving multiple mechanisms of direct and indirect action through D1Rs and D2Rs, affecting presynaptic release, NMDA, GABA, AMPA, Na^+, Ca^{2+}, and K^+ currents, among others. Various studies have reported either primarily inhibitory, excitatory, or heterogenous effects of DA on PFC neurons. The main points we wish to emphasize here are that DA acts as a neuromodulator, altering the efficacy of synaptic input to prefrontal neurons, and that there is some optimal level of DA-ergic stimulation for a neuron to experience, with greater or lesser DA signaling leading to an erosion of task related activity." (Clark & Noudoost, 2014)

"An individual's response to a given pharmacological manipulation of monoamine activity will vary depending on intrinsic monoamine levels." (Tipper et al., 2005)

"Psychostimulants such as Adderall are widely used for cognitive enhancement by healthy young people, yet laboratory research on effectiveness has yielded variable results. The present study assessed the effects of ADL in healthy young adults with an adequately powered double-blind cross-over placebo-controlled trial. We examined effects in 13 measures of cognitive ability including episodic memory, working memory, inhibitory control, convergent creativity, intelligence and scholastic achievement, with the goals of determining (1) whether the drug is at least moderately enhancing (Cohen's d >= .5) to some or all cognitive abilities tested, (2) whether its effects on cognition are moderated by baseline ability or COMT genotype, and (3) whether it induces an illusory perception of cognitive enhancement. The results did not reveal enhancement of any cognitive abilities by ADL for participants in general. There was a suggestion of moderation of enhancement by baseline ability and COMT genotype in a minority of tasks, with ADL enhancing *lower ability participants* on word recall, embedded figures and Raven's Progressive Matrices. Despite the lack of enhancement observed for most measures and most participants, participants nevertheless believed their performance was more enhanced by the active capsule than by placebo. We conclude that ADL has no more than small effects on cognition in healthy young adults, although users may perceive the drug as enhancing their cognition." (Ilieva et al., 2013)

65, p165. *The Inverted-U Theory*.

"Methylphenidate (Ritalin) is widely prescribed for hyperkinetic children. This study showed a peak enhancement of learning in children after being given a dose of 0.3 milligram per kilogram of body weight, and a decrement in learning in those given larger doses; social behavior showed the most improvement in children given 1.0 milligram per kilogram. These results had been hypothesized from theoretical dose-response curves which indicate different target behaviors would improve at different doses." (Sprague & Sleator, 1977)

66, p167. *Stimulants drugs keep those empty spaces closed.*

Stimulants suppress default mode activity: "We evaluated cortical activation differences in adults with ADHD before and after amphetamine medication in a demanding auditory attention task using MEG-based beamforming. Prior to psychostimulant medication, we observed neuronal desynchronization in the gamma-band frequency (68–88 Hz) in the medial prefrontal cortex which was reduced after psychostimulant administration. Such enhanced medial prefrontal cortex activity supports our original hypothesis and reflects improved suppression of default-mode activity." (Franzen & Wilson, 2012)

"Studies in non-ADHD adults suggest that stimulants do not promote acquisition of new information, might improve retention of previously acquired information, and facilitate memory consolidation, but may actually impair performance of tasks that require adaptation, flexibility and planning. It is still not clear if improvement only occurs when there is a baseline deficit. Stimulants may influence cognition by their effects on physiological arousal." (Advokat, 2010)

67, p167. *How can a smart pill degrade your cognitive performance?*

Neuroscientists can use single unit recordings to study neural dynamics during a task. The experiments are done in animals, with electrodes inserted into multiple neurons in a region where a task is processed. The monkey responds to the task – find the peanut under a cup. As his neurons fire, the electrodes trace a series of random patterns that eventually settle into a discrete activity pattern. That pattern is referred to as an *attractor* or an attractor network. Functions like remembering or moving happen because a neural network settles into an attractor. As the monkey executes the peanut test, he transitions from a memory attractor network to a response attractor. Attractor networks have different characteristics; stable or unstable, robust or weak, etc. Transitions among attractor states may be efficient or not, coherent or not, etc.

As it happens, amphetamine has differential effects on attractor dynamics depending on dose. Low doses promote the stability and coherence of attractor states while high doses are disruptive. Generating attractors and transitioning among them is the way computational neuroscientists talk about thought and behavior. It happens all the time, it's the way brain networks form and unform and, in the prefrontal cortex, it is regulated by the activity of norepinephrine and dopamine.

A working memory task is like this: *Say these numbers to me, backwards: 9673018.* The seven-digit number is captured in one's working memory as serial digits, in an attractor network. Then, a second attractor network forms because you have to repeat the number backwards. (The correct answer, BTW, is 8103769.) In monkeys, the nature of the working memory test is different, but the amphetamine effect is the same as it is in humans: an inverted U-shaped dose–response profile. With respect to working memory, performance is improved by low doses, whereas high doses impair performance.

"Animals treated with 1.0 mg/kg AMPH exhibited a clear separation of task epochs and ordered neural flow fields, whereas this organization completely broke down in animals treated with the 3.3 mg/kg dose of AMPH. With this higher dose, orbits corresponding to the different task phases could not be discerned, even in the optimally expanded space.

"Examining the second- and higher-order cross-correlations among units provides additional insights into what underlies the improved state space separation in the 1.0 mg AMPH group, in contrast to the diminished separation for the 3.3 mg AMPH group. Indeed, across the range of orders examined (orders 2–4), these rate correlations were always highest for the 1.0 mg AMPH group and always lowest for the 3.3 mg AMPH group. The fact that unit correlations at all orders examined were weak for the 3.3 mg AMPH group explains why expanding the neural state spaces does not help much in improving separation for this condition. Correlations and thus product terms in the basis expansion simply did not add any additional information that would help to separate trajectories for high AMPH or, even worse, may have added noise in this case. Thus, although after a low dose of AMPH network dynamics seem to become more coherent and coordinated, network dynamics appear to become mostly disorganized and incoherent when rats received the higher 3.3 mg/kg dose of AMPH." (Lapish et al., 2015)

68, p168. *The only existing molecules that reliably improve attention, memory and psychomotor speed.*

There are others, but their cognitive effects are not quite so robust nor so predictable. There are the non-stimulant ADD treatments: atomoxetine (Straterra) and viloxazine (Quelbree), which are not dissimilar to antidepressants that stimulate norepinephrine (bupropion, desipramine). Amantadine is an NMDA antagonist that may also stimulate dopamine, and is more potent than its close relative, memantine (Namenda), which is used in cases of early dementia. Modafanil and armodafinil (Nuvigil) are unique drugs that promote wakefulness without incurring a sleep debt. They are effective for ADD but were never submitted for FDA approval because of a serious side effect.

FINAL NOTE: The characters in this book were real patients at our clinics but identifying characteristics, like age, sex, occupation, etc., have been changed.

REFERENCES

Advokat, C. (2010). What are the cognitive effects of stimulant medications? Emphasis on adults with attention-deficit/hyperactivity disorder (ADHD). *Neuroscience & Biobehavioral Reviews*, *34*(8), 1256–1266. https://doi.org/10.1016/j.neubiorev.2010.03.006

Allport, G., & Odbert, H. (1936). *Trait Names A Psycho-lexical Study*. Psychological Review Company.

Alsherbiny, M. A., & Li, C. G. (2019). Medicinal Cannabis—Potential Drug Interactions. *Medicines*, *6*(1), Article 1. https://doi.org/10.3390/medicines6010003

Aman, M. G., Vamos, M., & Werry, J. S. (1984). Effects of Methylphenidate in Normal Adults with Reference to Drug Action in Hyperactivity. *Australian and New Zealand Journal of Psychiatry*, *18*(1), 86–88. https://doi.org/10.3109/00048678409161040

American Psychiatric Association (Ed.). (2022). *Diagnostic and statistical manual of mental disorders: DSM-V - Text Revision*.

Anderson, K. N., Dutton, A. C., Broussard, C. S., Farr, S. L., Lind, J. N., Visser, S. N., Ailes, E. C., Shapira, S. K., Reefhuis, J., & Tinker, S. C. (2020). ADHD Medication Use During Pregnancy and Risk for Selected Birth Defects: National Birth Defects Prevention Study, 1998-2011. *Journal of Attention Disorders*, *24*(3), 479–489. https://doi.org/10.1177/1087054718759753

Arendt, M., Munk-Jørgensen, P., Sher, L., & Jensen, S. O. W. (2011). Mortality among individuals with cannabis, cocaine, amphetamine, MDMA, and opioid use disorders: A nationwide follow-up study of Danish substance users in treatment. *Drug and Alcohol*

Dependence, *114*(2–3), 134–139.
https://doi.org/10.1016/j.drugalcdep.2010.09.013

Arria, A. M., Caldeira, K. M., O'Grady, K. E., Vincent, K. B., Johnson, E. P., & Wish, E. D. (2008). Nonmedical Use of Prescription Stimulants Among College Students: Associations with Attention-Deficit-Hyperactivity Disorder and Polydrug Use. *Pharmacotherapy: The Journal of Human Pharmacology and Drug Therapy, 28*(2), 156–169. https://doi.org/10.1592/phco.28.2.156

Barbaresi, W. J., Colligan, R. C., Weaver, A. L., Voigt, R. G., Killian, J. M., & Katusic, S. K. (2013). Mortality, ADHD, and Psychosocial Adversity in Adults With Childhood ADHD: A Prospective Study. *Pediatrics, 131*(4), 637–644. https://doi.org/10.1542/peds.2012-2354

Barbaresi, W. J., Katusic, S. K., Colligan, R. C., Pankratz, V. S., Weaver, A. L., Weber, K. J., Mrazek, D. A., & Jacobsen, S. J. (2002). How Common Is Attention-Deficit/Hyperactivity Disorder?: Incidence in a Population-Based Birth Cohort in Rochester, Minn. *Archives of Pediatrics & Adolescent Medicine, 156*(3), 217–224. https://doi.org/10.1001/archpedi.156.3.217

Barker, D. J. P. (1995). Fetal origins of coronary heart disease. *BMJ, 311*(6998), 171–174. https://doi.org/10.1136/bmj.311.6998.171

Barkley, R. A., Guevremont, D. C., Anastopoulos, A. D., DuPaul, G. J., & Shelton, T. L. (1993). Driving-Related Risks and Outcomes of Attention Deficit Hyperactivity Disorder in Adolescents and Young Adults: A 3- to 5-Year Follow-up Survey. *Pediatrics, 92*(2), 212–218. https://doi.org/10.1542/peds.92.2.212

Bax, M., & MacKeith, R. (1963). *Minimal Cerebral Dysfunction.* https://www.tiberbooks.com/product/91884/Minimal-Cerebral-Dysfunction--Little-Club-Clinics-in-Developmental-Medicine-No-10-Bax-Martin-and-Ronald-Mac-Keith-eds

Benes, F. M., Turtle, M., Khan, Y., & Farol, P. (1994). Myelination of a Key Relay Zone in the Hippocampal Formation

Occurs in the Human Brain During Childhood,
Adolescence, and Adulthood. *Archives of General
Psychiatry*, *51*(6), 477–484.
https://doi.org/10.1001/archpsyc.1994.0395006004100
4

Berner, S. (2007). Information Overload Or Attention
Deficiency? *Journal of Systems and Information
Technology*, 45–52.

Berridge, C. W. (2006). Neural Substrates of Psychostimulant-
Induced Arousal. *Neuropsychopharmacology*, *31*(11),
2332–2340. https://doi.org/10.1038/sj.npp.1301159

Besag, F. M. C. (2014). ADHD Treatment and Pregnancy. *Drug
Safety*, *37*(6), 397–408.
https://doi.org/10.1007/s40264-014-0168-5

Bishop, S., Duncan, J., Brett, M., & Lawrence, A. D. (2004).
Prefrontal cortical function and anxiety: Controlling
attention to threat-related stimuli. *Nature
Neuroscience*, *7*(2), 184–188.
https://doi.org/10.1038/nn1173

Bishop, S. J. (2009). Trait anxiety and impoverished prefrontal
control of attention. *Nature Neuroscience*, *12*(1), 92–98.
https://doi.org/10.1038/nn.2242

Blythe, P. (1979). MINIMAL BRAIN DYSFUNCTION AND THE
TREATMENT OF PSYCHONEUROSES. In M. Carruthers &
P. Mellett (Eds.), *The Coming Age of Psychosomatics*
(pp. 247–255). Pergamon.
https://doi.org/10.1016/B978-0-08-023736-7.50008-3

Bro, S. P., Kjaersgaard, M. I. S., Parner, E. T., Sørensen, M. J.,
Olsen, J., Bech, B. H., Pedersen, L. H., Christensen, J., &
Vestergaard, M. (2015). Adverse pregnancy outcomes
after exposure to methylphenidate or atomoxetine
during pregnancy. *Clinical Epidemiology*, *7*, 139–147.
https://doi.org/10.2147/CLEP.S72906

Broyd, S. J., Demanuele, C., Debener, S., Helps, S. K., James, C. J.,
& Sonuga-Barke, E. J. S. (2009). Default-mode brain
dysfunction in mental disorders: A systematic review.

Neuroscience & Biobehavioral Reviews, 33(3), 279–296.
https://doi.org/10.1016/j.neubiorev.2008.09.002

Buckner, R. L., Andrews-Hanna, J. R., & Schacter, D. L. (2008).
The brain's default network: Anatomy, function, and
relevance to disease. *Annals of the New York Academy
of Sciences, 1124*, 1–38.
https://doi.org/10.1196/annals.1440.011

Burgard, D. A., Fuller, R., Becker, B., Ferrell, R., & Dinglasan-
Panlilio, M. J. (2013). Potential trends in Attention
Deficit Hyperactivity Disorder (ADHD) drug use on a
college campus: Wastewater analysis of amphetamine
and ritalinic acid. *Science of the Total Environment, 450*,
242–249.

Cantu, C., Arauz, A., Murillo-Bonilla, L. M., López, M., &
Barinagarrementeria, F. (2003). Stroke Associated With
Sympathomimetics Contained in Over-the-Counter
Cough and Cold Drugs. *Stroke, 34*(7), 1667–1672.
https://doi.org/10.1161/01.STR.0000075293.45936.FA

Cattell, H. E. P., & Mead, A. D. (2008). The Sixteen Personality
Factor Questionnaire (16PF). In G. Boyle, G. Matthews,
& D. Saklofske, *The SAGE Handbook of Personality
Theory and Assessment: Volume 2—Personality
Measurement and Testing* (pp. 135–159). SAGE
Publications Ltd.
https://doi.org/10.4135/9781849200479.n7

Cattell, R. B. (1943). The description of personality: Basic traits
resolved into clusters. *The Journal of Abnormal and
Social Psychology, 38*(4), 476–506.
https://doi.org/10.1037/h0054116

Cattell, R. B. (1947). Confirmation and clarification of primary
personality factors. *Psychometrika, 12*(3), 197–220.
https://doi.org/10.1007/BF02289253

Chen, V. C.-H., Chan, H.-L., Wu, S.-I., Lee, M., Lu, M.-L., Liang, H.-
Y., Dewey, M. E., Stewart, R., & Lee, C. T.-C. (2019).
Attention-Deficit/Hyperactivity Disorder and Mortality
Risk in Taiwan. *JAMA Network Open, 2*(8), e198714.
https://doi.org/10.1001/jamanetworkopen.2019.8714

Clark, K. L., & Noudoost, B. (2014). The role of prefrontal
       catecholamines in attention and working memory.
       Frontiers in Neural Circuits, 8.
       https://www.frontiersin.org/articles/10.3389/fncir.2014
       .00033

Clemow, D. B., & Walker, D. J. (2014). The potential for misuse
       and abuse of medications in ADHD: A review.
       Postgraduate Medicine, 126(5), 64–81.
       https://doi.org/10.3810/pgm.2014.09.2801

Compton, W. M., Han, B., Blanco, C., Johnson, K., & Jones, C. M.
       (2018). Prevalence and correlates of prescription
       stimulant use, misuse, use disorders, and motivations
       for misuse among adults in the U.S. *The American
       Journal of Psychiatry, 175*(8), 741–755.
       https://doi.org/10.1176/appi.ajp.2018.17091048

Conner, S. N., Carter, E. B., Tuuli, M. G., Macones, G. A., & Cahill,
       A. G. (2015). Maternal marijuana use and neonatal
       morbidity. *American Journal of Obstetrics and
       Gynecology, 213*(3), 422.e1-4.
       https://doi.org/10.1016/j.ajog.2015.05.050

Conners, C. K., Eisenberg, L., & Barcai, A. (1967). Effect of
       Dextroamphetamine on Children: Studies on Subjects
       With Learning Disabilities and School Behavior
       Problems. *Archives of General Psychiatry, 17*(4), 478–
       485.
       https://doi.org/10.1001/archpsyc.1967.0173028009401
       1

Cooper, M., Thapar, A., & Jones, D. K. (2015). ADHD severity is
       associated with white matter microstructure in the
       subgenual cingulum. NeuroImage☐:*Clinical, 7*, 653–660.
       https://doi.org/10.1016/j.nicl.2015.02.012

Cox, D. J., Merkel, R. L., Moore, M., Thorndike, F., Muller, C., &
       Kovatchev, B. (2006). Relative Benefits of Stimulant
       Therapy With OROS Methylphenidate Versus Mixed
       Amphetamine Salts Extended Release in Improving the
       Driving Performance of Adolescent Drivers With
       Attention-Deficit/Hyperactivity Disorder. *Pediatrics,*

118(3), e704–e710. https://doi.org/10.1542/peds.2005-2947

Daldegan-Bueno, D., Maia, L. O., Glass, M., Jutras-Aswad, D., & Fischer, B. (2022). Co-exposure of cannabinoids with amphetamines and biological, behavioural and health outcomes: A scoping review of animal and human studies. *Psychopharmacology, 239*(5), 1211–1230. https://doi.org/10.1007/s00213-021-05960-2

Dalsgaard, S., Østergaard, S. D., Leckman, J. F., Mortensen, P. B., & Pedersen, M. G. (2015). Mortality in children, adolescents, and adults with attention deficit hyperactivity disorder: A nationwide cohort study. *The Lancet, 385*(9983), 2190–2196. https://doi.org/10.1016/S0140-6736(14)61684-6

Danielson, M. L. (2023). Trends in Stimulant Prescription Fills Among Commercially Insured Children and Adults—United States, 2016–2021. *MMWR. Morbidity and Mortality Weekly Report, 72*. https://doi.org/10.15585/mmwr.mm7213a1

Danielson, M. L., Bitsko, R. H., Ghandour, R. M., Holbrook, J. R., Kogan, M. D., & Blumberg, S. J. (2018). Prevalence of Parent-Reported ADHD Diagnosis and Associated Treatment Among U.S. Children and Adolescents, 2016. *Journal of Clinical Child and Adolescent Psychology: The Official Journal for the Society of Clinical Child and Adolescent Psychology, American Psychological Association, Division 53, 47*(2), 199–212. https://doi.org/10.1080/15374416.2017.1417860

Davies, I. (1939). Benzedrine: Uses and Abuses. *Proceedings of the Royal Society of Medicine, 32*(4), 385–398.

Dideriksen, D., Pottegård, A., Hallas, J., Aagaard, L., & Damkier, P. (2013). First trimester in utero exposure to methylphenidate. *Basic & Clinical Pharmacology & Toxicology, 112*(2), 73–76. https://doi.org/10.1111/bcpt.12034

Ding, M., Bhupathiraju, S. N., Satija, A., van Dam, R. M., & Hu, F. B. (2014). Long-term coffee consumption and risk of cardiovascular disease: A systematic review and a dose-response meta-analysis of prospective cohort studies. *Circulation, 129*(6), 643–659. https://doi.org/10.1161/CIRCULATIONAHA.113.005925

Dreher, M. C. (1984). Schoolchildren and Ganja: Youthful Marijuana Consumption in Rural Jamaica. *Anthropology & Education Quarterly, 15*(2), 131–150. https://doi.org/10.1525/aeq.1984.15.2.04x0470b

Du, J., Wang, Y., Hunter, R., Wei, Y., Blumenthal, R., Falke, C., Khairova, R., Zhou, R., Yuan, P., Machado-Vieira, R., McEwen, B. S., & Manji, H. K. (2009). Dynamic regulation of mitochondrial function by glucocorticoids. *Proceedings of the National Academy of Sciences, 106*(9), 3543–3548. https://doi.org/10.1073/pnas.0812671106

El Marroun, H., Tiemeier, H., Steegers, E. A. P., Jaddoe, V. W. V., Hofman, A., Verhulst, F. C., van den Brink, W., & Huizink, A. C. (2009). Intrauterine Cannabis Exposure Affects Fetal Growth Trajectories: The Generation R Study. *Journal of the American Academy of Child & Adolescent Psychiatry, 48*(12), 1173–1181. https://doi.org/10.1097/CHI.0b013e3181bfa8ee

Emanuel, R. M., Frellsen, S. L., Kashima, K. J., Sanguino, S. M., Sierles, F. S., & Lazarus, C. J. (2013). Cognitive Enhancement Drug Use Among Future Physicians: Findings from a Multi-Institutional Census of Medical Students. *Journal of General Internal Medicine, 28*(8), 1028–1034. https://doi.org/10.1007/s11606-012-2249-4

Eskelinen, M. H., & Kivipelto, M. (2010). Caffeine as a protective factor in dementia and Alzheimer's disease. *Journal of Alzheimer's Disease: JAD, 20 Suppl 1*, S167-174. https://doi.org/10.3233/JAD-2010-1404

Esteller-Cucala, P., Maceda, I., Børglum, A. D., Demontis, D., Faraone, S. V., Cormand, B., & Lao, O. (2020). Genomic analysis of the natural history of attention-deficit/hyperactivity disorder using Neanderthal and ancient Homo sapiens samples. *Scientific Reports, 10,* 8622. https://doi.org/10.1038/s41598-020-65322-4

Evans, M. A., Martz, R., Rodda, B. E., Lemberger, L., & Forney, R. B. (1976). Effects of marihuana-dextroamphetamine combination. *Clinical Pharmacology & Therapeutics, 20*(3), 350–358. https://doi.org/10.1002/cpt1976203350

Evans, R. W., Gualtieri, C. T., & Amara, I. (1986). Methylphenidate and memory: Dissociated effects in hyperactive children. *Psychopharmacology, 90*(2), 211–216.

Evans, R. W., Gualtieri, C. T., & Hicks, R. E. (1986). A neuropathic substrate for stimulant drug effects in hyperactive children. *Clinical Neuropharmacology, 9*(3), 264–281. https://doi.org/10.1097/00002826-198606000-00005

Eysenck, H. (1950). *Dimensions of Personality.* Routledge & Kegan Paul limited. http://archive.org/details/dimensionsofpers0000hjey_e0a7

Eysenck, M. W., Derakshan, N., Santos, R., & Calvo, M. G. (2007). Anxiety and cognitive performance: Attentional control theory. *Emotion, 7*(2), 336–353. https://doi.org/10.1037/1528-3542.7.2.336

Faraone, S. V., & Biederman, J. (2005). What Is the Prevalence of Adult ADHD? Results of a Population Screen of 966 Adults. *Journal of Attention Disorders, 9*(2), 384–391. https://doi.org/10.1177/1087054705281478

Ferrucci, M., Limanaqi, F., Ryskalin, L., Biagioni, F., Busceti, C. L., & Fornai, F. (2019). The Effects of Amphetamine and Methamphetamine on the Release of Norepinephrine, Dopamine and Acetylcholine From the Brainstem Reticular Formation. *Frontiers in Neuroanatomy, 13,* 48. https://doi.org/10.3389/fnana.2019.00048

Filiou, M. D., & Sandi, C. (2019). Anxiety and Brain Mitochondria: A Bidirectional Crosstalk. *Trends in Neurosciences, 42*(9), 573–588. https://doi.org/10.1016/j.tins.2019.07.002

Finger, G., Silva, E. R. da, & Falavigna, A. (2013). Use of methylphenidate among medical students: A systematic review. *Revista Da Associação Médica Brasileira*, *59*(3), 285–289. https://doi.org/10.1016/j.ramb.2012.10.007

Flory, C. D., & Gilbert, J. (1943). The effects of benzedrine sulphate and caffeine citrate on the efficiency of college students. *Journal of Applied Psychology*, *27*(2), 121–134. https://doi.org/10.1037/h0060179

Franke, B., Michelini, G., Asherson, P., Banaschewski, T., Bilbow, A., Buitelaar, J. K., Cormand, B., Faraone, S. V., Ginsberg, Y., Haavik, J., Kuntsi, J., Larsson, H., Lesch, K.-P., Ramos-Quiroga, J. A., Réthelyi, J. M., Ribases, M., & Reif, A. (2018). Live fast, die young? A review on the developmental trajectories of ADHD across the lifespan. *European Neuropsychopharmacology*, *28*(10), 1059–1088. https://doi.org/10.1016/j.euroneuro.2018.08.001

Franzen, J. D., & Wilson, T. W. (2012). Amphetamines Modulate Prefrontal Gamma Oscillations during Attention Processing. *Neuroreport*, *23*(12), 731–735. https://doi.org/10.1097/WNR.0b013e328356bb59

Gajewski, K. K., & Saul, J. P. (2010). Sudden cardiac death in children and adolescents (excluding Sudden Infant Death Syndrome). *Annals of Pediatric Cardiology*, *3*(2), 107–112. https://doi.org/10.4103/0974-2069.74035

Gallucci, A. R., Martin, R. J., & Usdan, S. L. (2015). The diversion of stimulant medications among a convenience sample of college students with current prescriptions. *Psychology of Addictive Behaviors: Journal of the Society of Psychologists in Addictive Behaviors*, *29*(1), 154–161. https://doi.org/10.1037/adb0000012

Garnier, L. M., Arria, A. M., Caldeira, K. M., Vincent, K. B., O'Grady, K. E., & Wish, E. D. (2010). Sharing and selling of prescription medications in a college student sample. *The Journal of Clinical Psychiatry*, *71*(3), 262–269. https://doi.org/10.4088/JCP.09m05189ecr

Ghassemzadeh, H., Rothbart, M. K., & Posner, M. I. (2019). Anxiety and Brain Networks of Attentional Control.

Cognitive and Behavioral Neurology, *32*(1), 54–62.
https://doi.org/10.1097/WNN.0000000000000181

Gillberg, C., & Kadesjö, B. (2003). Why bother about clumsiness? The implications of having developmental coordination disorder (DCD). *Neural Plasticity*, *10*(1–2), 59–68.

Good, M. M., Solt, I., Acuna, J. G., Rotmensch, S., & Kim, M. J. (2010). Methamphetamine Use During Pregnancy: Maternal and Neonatal Implications. *Obstetrics & Gynecology*, *116*(2 Part 1), 330–334.
https://doi.org/10.1097/AOG.0b013e3181e67094

Graham, P., & Rutter, M. (1968). Organic Brain Dysfunction and Child Psychiatric Disorder. *BMJ*, *3*(5620), 695–700.
https://doi.org/10.1136/bmj.3.5620.695

Grant, K. S., Petroff, R., Isoherranen, N., Stella, N., & Burbacher, T. M. (2018). Cannabis Use during Pregnancy: Pharmacokinetics and Effects on Child Development. *Pharmacology & Therapeutics*, *182*, 133–151.
https://doi.org/10.1016/j.pharmthera.2017.08.014

Greely, H., Sahakian, B., Harris, J., Kessler, R. C., Gazzaniga, M., Campbell, P., & Farah, M. J. (2008). Towards responsible use of cognitive-enhancing drugs by the healthy. *Nature*, *456*(7223), Article 7223.
https://doi.org/10.1038/456702a

Grosso, G., Godos, J., Galvano, F., & Giovannucci, E. L. (2017). Coffee, Caffeine, and Health Outcomes: An Umbrella Review. *Annual Review of Nutrition*, *37*, 131–156.
https://doi.org/10.1146/annurev-nutr-071816-064941

Gualtieri, C., & Johnson, L. (2006). Efficient allocation of attentional resources in patients with ADHD: Maturational changes from age 10 to 29. *Journal of Attention Disorders*, *9*(3), 534–542.
https://doi.org/10.1177/1087054705283758

Gualtieri, C., & Morgan, D. (2008). The frequency of cognitive impairment in patients with anxiety, depression, and bipolar disorder: An unaccounted source of variance in clinical trials. *The Journal of Clinical Psychiatry*, *69*(7), 1122–1130.

Gualtieri, C. T. (2021). Genomic Variation, Evolvability, and the Paradox of Mental Illness. *Frontiers in Psychiatry, 0.* https://doi.org/10.3389/fpsyt.2020.593233

Gualtieri, C. T., Adams, A., Shen, C. D., & Loiselle, D. (1982). Minor physical anomalies in alcoholic and schizophrenic adults and hyperactive and autistic children. *The American Journal of Psychiatry.* http://psycnet.apa.org/psycinfo/1982-23619-001

Gualtieri, C. T., & Hicks, R. E. (1985). Neuropharmacology of Methylphenidate and a Neural Substrate for Childhood Hyperactivity. *Psychiatric Clinics of North America, 8*(4), 875–892. https://doi.org/10.1016/S0193-953X(18)30661-0

Gualtieri, C. T., Hicks, R. E., & Mayo, J. P. (1983). Hyperactivity and Homeostasis. *Journal of the American Academy of Child Psychiatry, 22*(4), 382–384. https://doi.org/10.1016/S0002-7138(09)60677-4

Gualtieri, C. T., Ondrusek, M. G., & Finley, C. (1985). Attention Deficit Disorders in Adults. *Clinical Neuropharmacology, 8*(4), 343.

Gualtieri, C. T., Quade, D., Hicks, R. E., Mayo, J. P., & Schroeder, S. R. (1984). Tardive dyskinesia and other clinical consequences of neuroleptic treatment in children and adolescents. *The American Journal of Psychiatry, 141*(1), 20–23. https://doi.org/10.1176/ajp.141.1.20

Gunn, J. K. L., Rosales, C. B., Center, K. E., Nuñez, A., Gibson, S. J., Christ, C., & Ehiri, J. E. (2016). Prenatal exposure to cannabis and maternal and child health outcomes: A systematic review and meta-analysis. *BMJ Open, 6*(4), e009986. https://doi.org/10.1136/bmjopen-2015-009986

Hallowell, E., & Ratey, J. J. R. (2013). *Answers to Distraction.* Knopf Doubleday Publishing Group.

Hayatbakhsh, M. R., Flenady, V. J., Gibbons, K. S., Kingsbury, A. M., Hurrion, E., Mamun, A. A., & Najman, J. M. (2012). Birth outcomes associated with cannabis use before and during pregnancy. *Pediatric Research, 71*(2), Article 2. https://doi.org/10.1038/pr.2011.25

Hoogman, M., Bralten, J., Hibar, D. P., Mennes, M., Zwiers, M. P., Schweren, L. S. J., Hulzen, K. J. E. van, Medland, S. E., Shumskaya, E., Jahanshad, N., Zeeuw, P. de, Szekely, E., Sudre, G., Wolfers, T., Onnink, A. M. H., Dammers, J. T., Mostert, J. C., Vives-Gilabert, Y., Kohls, G., ... Franke, B. (2017). Subcortical brain volume differences in participants with attention deficit hyperactivity disorder in children and adults: A cross-sectional mega-analysis. *The Lancet Psychiatry, 4*(4), 310–319. https://doi.org/10.1016/S2215-0366(17)30049-4

Hou, J., Song, L., Zhang, W., Wu, W., Wang, J., Zhou, D., Qu, W., Guo, J., Gu, S., He, M., Xie, B., & Li, H. (2013). Morphologic and functional connectivity alterations of corticostriatal and default mode network in treatment-naïve patients with obsessive-compulsive disorder. *PloS One, 8*(12), e83931. https://doi.org/10.1371/journal.pone.0083931

Hubert, G. W., Jones, D. C., Moffett, M. C., Rogge, G., & Kuhar, M. J. (2008). CART Peptides as Modulators of Dopamine and Psychostimulants and Interactions with the Mesolimbic Dopaminergic System. *Biochemical Pharmacology, 75*(1), 57–62. https://doi.org/10.1016/j.bcp.2007.07.028

Huybrechts, K. F., Bröms, G., Christensen, L. B., Einarsdóttir, K., Engeland, A., Furu, K., Gissler, M., Hernandez-Diaz, S., Karlsson, P., Karlstad, Ø., Kieler, H., Lahesmaa-Korpinen, A.-M., Mogun, H., Nørgaard, M., Reutfors, J., Sørensen, H. T., Zoega, H., & Bateman, B. T. (2018). Association Between Methylphenidate and Amphetamine Use in Pregnancy and Risk of Congenital Malformations: A Cohort Study From the International Pregnancy Safety Study Consortium. *JAMA Psychiatry, 75*(2), 167–175. https://doi.org/10.1001/jamapsychiatry.2017.3644

Ilieva, I., Boland, J., & Farah, M. J. (2013). Objective and subjective cognitive enhancing effects of mixed amphetamine salts in healthy people. *Neuropharmacology, 64*, 496–505. https://doi.org/10.1016/j.neuropharm.2012.07.021

Ingvar, D. H. (1979). "Hyperfrontal" distribution of the cerebral grey matter flow in resting wakefulness; on the functional anatomy of the conscious state. *Acta Neurologica Scandinavica, 60*(1), 12–25. https://doi.org/10.1111/j.1600-0404.1979.tb02947.x

Jaques, S. C., Kingsbury, A., Henshcke, P., Chomchai, C., Clews, S., Falconer, J., Abdel-Latif, M. E., Feller, J. M., & Oei, J. L. (2014). Cannabis, the pregnant woman and her child: Weeding out the myths. *Journal of Perinatology, 34*(6), Article 6. https://doi.org/10.1038/jp.2013.180

Jensen, P. S., Mrazek, D., Knapp, P. K., Steinberg, L., Pfeffer, C., Schowalter, J., & Shapiro, T. (1997). Evolution and Revolution in Child Psychiatry: ADHD as a Disorder of Adaptation. *Journal of the American Academy of Child & Adolescent Psychiatry, 36*(12), 1672–1681. https://doi.org/10.1097/00004583-199712000-00015

Jones, P. B. (2013). Adult mental health disorders and their age at onset. *British Journal of Psychiatry, 202*(s54), s5–s10. https://doi.org/10.1192/bjp.bp.112.119164

Katzman, M. A., Bilkey, T. S., Chokka, P. R., Fallu, A., & Klassen, L. J. (2017). Adult ADHD and comorbid disorders: Clinical implications of a dimensional approach. *BMC Psychiatry, 17*(1), 302. https://doi.org/10.1186/s12888-017-1463-3

Klein, R. G., Mannuzza, S., Olazagasti, M. A. R., Roizen, E., Hutchison, J. A., Lashua, E. C., & Castellanos, F. X. (2012). Clinical and Functional Outcome of Childhood Attention-Deficit/Hyperactivity Disorder 33 Years Later. *Archives of General Psychiatry, 69*(12), 1295–1303. https://doi.org/10.1001/archgenpsychiatry.2012.271

Knouse, L. E., Traeger, L., O'Cleirigh, C., & Safren, S. A. (2013). Adult ADHD Symptoms and Five Factor Model Traits in a Clinical Sample: A Structural Equation Modeling Approach. *The Journal of Nervous and Mental Disease,*

201(10), 10.1097/NMD.0b013e3182a5bf33.
https://doi.org/10.1097/NMD.0b013e3182a5bf33

Kolding, L., Ehrenstein, V., Pedersen, L., Sandager, P., Petersen, O. B., Uldbjerg, N., & Pedersen, L. H. (2021). Associations Between ADHD Medication Use in Pregnancy and Severe Malformations Based on Prenatal and Postnatal Diagnoses: A Danish Registry-Based Study. *The Journal of Clinical Psychiatry, 82*(1), 20m13458. https://doi.org/10.4088/JCP.20m13458

Koren, G., Barer, Y., & Ornoy, A. (2020). Fetal safety of methylphenidate—A scoping review and meta analysis. *Reproductive Toxicology, 93*, 230–234. https://doi.org/10.1016/j.reprotox.2020.03.003

Koutsoklenis, A., & Honkasilta, J. (2023). ADHD in the DSM-5-TR: What has changed and what has not. *Frontiers in Psychiatry, 13*. https://www.frontiersin.org/articles/10.3389/fpsyt.2022.1064141

Kumer, S. C., & Vrana, K. E. (1996). Intricate Regulation of Tyrosine Hydroxylase Activity and Gene Expression. *Journal of Neurochemistry, 67*(2), 443–462. https://doi.org/10.1046/j.1471-4159.1996.67020443.x

Ladhani, N. N. N., Shah, P. S., & Murphy, K. E. (2011). Prenatal amphetamine exposure and birth outcomes: A systematic review and metaanalysis. *American Journal of Obstetrics and Gynecology, 205*(3), 219.e1-219.e7. https://doi.org/10.1016/j.ajog.2011.04.016

Lapish, C. C., Balaguer-Ballester, E., Seamans, J. K., Phillips, A. G., & Durstewitz, D. (2015). Amphetamine Exerts Dose-Dependent Changes in Prefrontal Cortex Attractor Dynamics during Working Memory. *Journal of Neuroscience, 35*(28), 10172–10187. https://doi.org/10.1523/JNEUROSCI.2421-14.2015

Lapouse, R., & Monk, M. A. (1958). An epidemiologic study of behavior characteristics in children. *American Journal of Public Health and the Nation's Health, 48*(9), 1134–1144.

Latronica, J. R., Clegg, T. J., Tuan, W.-J., & Bone, C. (2021). Are Amphetamines Associated with Adverse Cardiovascular Events Among Elderly Individuals? *The Journal of the American Board of Family Medicine, 34*(6), 1074–1081. https://doi.org/10.3122/jabfm.2021.06.210228

Laufer, M. W., Denhoff, E., & Solomons, G. (1957). Hyperkinetic Impulse Disorder in Children's Behavior Problems. *Journal of Attention Disorders, 15*(8), 620–625. https://doi.org/10.1177/1087054711413043

Lee, M., McGeer, E. G., & McGeer, P. L. (2016). Quercetin, not caffeine, is a major neuroprotective component in coffee. *Neurobiology of Aging, 46*, 113–123. https://doi.org/10.1016/j.neurobiolaging.2016.06.015

Liu, Y.-C., Chen, V. C.-H., Yang, Y.-H., Chen, Y.-L., & Gossop, M. (2021). Association of psychiatric comorbidities with the risk of transport accidents in ADHD and MPH. *Epidemiology and Psychiatric Sciences, 30*. https://doi.org/10.1017/S2045796021000032

London, A. S., & Landes, S. D. (2016). Attention Deficit Hyperactivity Disorder and adult mortality. *Preventive Medicine, 90*, 8–10. https://doi.org/10.1016/j.ypmed.2016.06.021

Louik, C., Kerr, S., Kelley, K. E., & Mitchell, A. A. (2015). Increasing Use of ADHD Medications in Pregnancy. *Pharmacoepidemiology and Drug Safety, 24*(2), 218–220. https://doi.org/10.1002/pds.3742

Maher, B. (2008). Poll results: Look who's doping. *Nature, 452*(7188), 674–675. https://doi.org/10.1038/452674a

Markowitz, J., & Patrick, K. (2005). Pharmacokinetic and Pharmacodynamic Drug Interactions: Methylphenidate, Amphetamine or Atomoxetine in Attention Deficit Hyperactivity Disorder . In *ATTENTION DEFICIT HYPERACTIVITY DISORDER From Genes to Patients* (pp. 529–550). Humana Press.

Martel, M. M., Nigg, J. T., & von Eye, A. (2008). How Do Trait Dimensions Map onto ADHD Symptom Domains?

Journal of Abnormal Child Psychology, 37(3), 337.
https://doi.org/10.1007/s10802-008-9255-3

McCabe, S. E., & Boyd, C. J. (2005). Sources of prescription drugs for illicit use. *Addictive Behaviors, 30*(7), 1342–1350. https://doi.org/10.1016/j.addbeh.2005.01.012

McCabe, S. E., Knight, J. R., Teter, C. J., & Wechsler, H. (2005). Non-medical use of prescription stimulants among US college students: Prevalence and correlates from a national survey. *Addiction, 100*(1), 96–106. https://doi.org/10.1111/j.1360-0443.2005.00944.x

McCabe, S. E., Teter, C. J., & Boyd, C. J. (2004). The Use, Misuse and Diversion of Prescription Stimulants Among Middle and High School Students. *Substance Use & Misuse, 39*(7), 1095–1116. https://doi.org/10.1081/JA-120038031

McCabe, S. E., Teter, C. J., & Boyd, C. J. (2006). Medical Use, Illicit Use and Diversion of Prescription Stimulant Medication. *Journal of Psychoactive Drugs, 38*(1), 43–56.

McGaugh, J. L. (2000). Memory—A Century of Consolidation. *Science, 287*(5451), 248–251. https://doi.org/10.1126/science.287.5451.248

McKetin, R., Leung, J., Stockings, E., Huo, Y., Foulds, J., Lappin, J. M., Cumming, C., Arunogiri, S., Young, J. T., Sara, G., Farrell, M., & Degenhardt, L. (2019). Mental health outcomes associated with the use of amphetamines: A systematic review and meta-analysis. *EClinicalMedicine, 16*, 81–97. https://doi.org/10.1016/j.eclinm.2019.09.014

Metz, T. D., & Stickrath, E. H. (2015). Marijuana use in pregnancy and lactation: A review of the evidence. *American Journal of Obstetrics and Gynecology, 213*(6), 761–778. https://doi.org/10.1016/j.ajog.2015.05.025

Miller, C. J., Miller, S. R., Newcorn, J. H., & Halperin, J. M. (2008). Personality Characteristics Associated with Persistent ADHD in Late Adolescence. *Journal of Abnormal Child*

Psychology, 36(2), 165–173.
https://doi.org/10.1007/s10802-007-9167-7

Minkowsky, W. L. (1939). The effect of benzedrine sulphate upon learning. *Journal of Comparative Psychology, 28*(3), 349–360. https://doi.org/10.1037/h0060699

Minnes, S., Lang, A., & Singer, L. (2011). Prenatal Tobacco, Marijuana, Stimulant, and Opiate Exposure: Outcomes and Practice Implications. *Addiction Science & Clinical Practice, 6*(1), 57–70.

Mogg, K., McNamara, J., Powys, M., Rawlinson, H., Seiffer, A., & Bradley, B. P. (2000). Selective attention to threat: A test of two cognitive models of anxiety. *Cognition & Emotion, 14*(3), 375–399.
https://doi.org/10.1080/026999300378888

Molitch, M., & Eccles, A. K. (1937). The effect of benzedrine sulfate on the intelligence scores of children. *American Journal of Psychiatry, 94*(3), 587–590.
https://doi.org/10.1176/ajp.94.3.587

Moore, D. R., Burgard, D. A., Larson, R. G., & Ferm, M. (2014). Psychostimulant use among college students during periods of high and low stress: An interdisciplinary approach utilizing both self-report and unobtrusive chemical sample data. *Addictive Behaviors, 39*(5), 987–993. https://doi.org/10.1016/j.addbeh.2014.01.021

Moore, T. J., Wirtz, P. W., Curran, J. N., & Alexander, G. C. (2023). Medical use and combination drug therapy among US adult users of central nervous system stimulants: A cross-sectional analysis. *BMJ Open, 13*(4), e069668. https://doi.org/10.1136/bmjopen-2022-069668

Moran, L. V., Ongur, D., Hsu, J., Castro, V. M., Perlis, R. H., & Schneeweiss, S. (2019). Psychosis with Methylphenidate or Amphetamine in Patients with ADHD. *New England Journal of Medicine, 380*(12), 1128–1138.
https://doi.org/10.1056/NEJMoa1813751

Moreno-Küstner, B., Martín, C., & Pastor, L. (2018). Prevalence of psychotic disorders and its association with methodological issues. A systematic review and meta-analyses. *PLoS ONE, 13*(4), e0195687. https://doi.org/10.1371/journal.pone.0195687

Morillo, C. A., Banerjee, A., Perel, P., Wood, D., & Jouven, X. (2017). Atrial fibrillation: The current epidemic. *Journal of Geriatric Cardiology⬜JGC, 14*(3), 195–203. https://doi.org/10.11909/j.issn.1671-5411.2017.03.011

Mosholder, A. D., Taylor, L., Mannheim, G., Ortendahl, L., Woodworth, T. S., & Toh, S. (2018). Incidence of Heart Failure and Cardiomyopathy Following Initiation of Medications for Attention-Deficit/Hyperactivity Disorder: A Descriptive Study. *Journal of Clinical Psychopharmacology, 38*(5), 505–508. https://doi.org/10.1097/JCP.0000000000000939

Muller, M., Sigurdsson, S., Kjartansson, O., Gunnarsdottir, I., Thorsdottir, I., Harris, T. B., van Buchem, M., Gudnason, V., Launer, L. J., & Age, Gene/Environment Susceptibility-Reykjavik Study Investigators. (2016). Late-life brain volume: A life-course approach. The AGES-Reykjavik study. *Neurobiology of Aging, 41*, 86–92. https://doi.org/10.1016/j.neurobiolaging.2016.02.012

Neelam, K., Garg, D., & Marshall, M. (2011). A systematic review and meta-analysis of neurological soft signs in relatives of people with schizophrenia. *BMC Psychiatry, 11*(1), 139.

Nigg, J. T., John, O. P., Blaskey, L. G., Huang-Pollock, C. L., Willcutt, E. G., Hinshaw, S. P., & Pennington, B. (2002). Big Five dimensions and ADHD symptoms: Links between personality traits and clinical symptoms. *Journal of Personality and Social Psychology, 83*(2), 451–469. https://doi.org/10.1037/0022-3514.83.2.451

Nissen, S. E. (2006). ADHD Drugs and Cardiovascular Risk. *New England Journal of Medicine, 354*(14), 1445–1448. https://doi.org/10.1056/NEJMp068049

Nörby, U., Winbladh, B., & Källén, K. (2017). Perinatal Outcomes After Treatment With ADHD Medication During

Pregnancy. *Pediatrics, 140*(6).
https://doi.org/10.1542/peds.2017-0747

O'Connor, M. (2018). Medicinal Cannabis in Pregnancy—
Panacea or Noxious Weed? *Journal of Law and
Medicine, 25*(3), 634–646.

Ornoy, A. (2018). Pharmacological Treatment of Attention
Deficit Hyperactivity Disorder During Pregnancy and
Lactation. *Pharmaceutical Research, 35*(3), 46.
https://doi.org/10.1007/s11095-017-2323-z

Ozgen, H. M., Hop, J. W., Hox, J. J., Beemer, F. A., & van
Engeland, H. (2008). Minor physical anomalies in
autism: A meta-analysis. *Molecular Psychiatry, 15*(3),
300–307. https://doi.org/10.1038/mp.2008.75

Parker, J. D. A., Majeski, S. A., & Collin, V. T. (2004). ADHD
symptoms and personality: Relationships with the five-
factor model. *Personality and Individual Differences,
36*(4), 977–987. https://doi.org/10.1016/S0191-
8869(03)00166-1

Patel, R. S., Manocha, P., Patel, J., Patel, R., & Tankersley, W. E.
(2020). Cannabis Use Is an Independent Predictor for
Acute Myocardial Infarction Related Hospitalization in
Younger Population. *Journal of Adolescent Health,
66*(1), 79–85.
https://doi.org/10.1016/j.jadohealth.2019.07.024

Perrin, J. M., Friedman, R. A., Knilans, T. K., the Black Box
Working Group, & the Section on Cardiology and
Cardiac Surgery. (2008). Cardiovascular Monitoring and
Stimulant Drugs for Attention-Deficit/Hyperactivity
Disorder. *Pediatrics, 122*(2), 451–453.
https://doi.org/10.1542/peds.2008-1573

Petersen, R. C. (1980). *Marijuana Research Findings, 1980.*
Department of Health and Human Services, Public
Health Service, Alcohol, Drug Abuse, and Mental Health
Administration, National Institute on Drug Abuse,
Division of Research.

Peterson, A., Thome, J., Frewen, P., & Lanius, R. A. (2014).
Resting-state neuroimaging studies: A new way of

identifying differences and similarities among the anxiety disorders? *Canadian Journal of Psychiatry. Revue Canadienne De Psychiatrie, 59*(6), 294–300.

Polanczyk, G., de Lima, M. S., Horta, B. L., Biederman, J., & Rohde, L. A. (2007). The Worldwide Prevalence of ADHD: A Systematic Review and Metaregression Analysis. *American Journal of Psychiatry, 164*(6), 942–948. https://doi.org/10.1176/ajp.2007.164.6.942

Raichle, M. E. (2010). Two views of brain function. *Trends in Cognitive Sciences, 14*(4), 180–190. https://doi.org/10.1016/j.tics.2010.01.008

Raman, S. R., Man, K. K., Bahmanyar, S., Berard, A., Bilder10, S., Boukhris, T., Bushnell11, G., Crystal10, S., Furu12, K., & KaoYang13, Y.-H. (2018). Regional and national trends in attention-deficit/hyperactivity disorder (ADHD) medication use: A multinational study in North America, Europe, Asia and Australia. *Lancet Psychiatry.*

Rapoport, J., Buchsbaum, M., Zahn, T., Weingartner, H., Ludlow, C., & Mikkelsen, E. (1978). Dextroamphetamine: Cognitive and behavioral effects in normal prepubertal boys. *Science, 199*(4328), 560–563. https://doi.org/10.1126/science.341313

Rasmussen, N. (2008). America's First Amphetamine Epidemic 1929–1971. *American Journal of Public Health, 98*(6), 974–985. https://doi.org/10.2105/AJPH.2007.110593

Redelmeier, D. A., Chan, W. K., & Lu, H. (2010). Road Trauma in Teenage Male Youth with Childhood Disruptive Behavior Disorders: A Population Based Analysis. *PLOS Medicine, 7*(11), e1000369. https://doi.org/10.1371/journal.pmed.1000369

Rowland, A. S., Skipper, B. J., Umbach, D. M., Rabiner, D. L., Campbell, R. A., Naftel, A. J., & Sandler, D. P. (2015). The Prevalence of ADHD in a Population-Based Sample. *Journal of Attention Disorders, 19*(9), 741–754. https://doi.org/10.1177/1087054713513799

Rutter, M. (1970). Psycho-Social Disorders in Childhood, and Their Outcome in Adult Life. *J Roy Coll Physicians London*, *4*(3), 211–219.

Rutter, M., & Graham, P. (1966). *Two Surveys of Children [Abridged] Psychiatric Disorder in 10-and 11-Year-Old Children*. SAGE Publications.

Safer, D. J. (2016). Recent Trends in Stimulant Usage. *Journal of Attention Disorders*, *20*(6), 471–477. https://doi.org/10.1177/1087054715605915

Safer, D. J. (2018). Is ADHD Really Increasing in Youth? *Journal of Attention Disorders*, *22*(2), 107–115. https://doi.org/10.1177/1087054715586571

Safer, D. J., & Krager, J. M. (1988). A survey of medication treatment for hyperactive/inattentive students. *JAMA*, *260*(15), 2256–2258.

Sargent, W. (1936). The effect of benzedrine on intelligence scores. *The Lancet*, *228*, 1385–1387. https://doi.org/10.1016/S0140-6736(00)75148-8

Sassi, K. L. M., Rocha, N. P., Colpo, G. D., John, V., & Teixeira, A. L. (2020). Amphetamine Use in the Elderly: A Systematic Review of the Literature. *Current Neuropharmacology*, *18*(2), 126–135. https://doi.org/10.2174/1570159X17666191010093021

Sayal, K., Prasad, V., Daley, D., Ford, T., & Coghill, D. (2018). ADHD in children and young people: Prevalence, care pathways, and service provision. *The Lancet. Psychiatry*, *5*(2), 175–186. https://doi.org/10.1016/S2215-0366(17)30167-0

Simon, V., Czobor, P., Bálint, S., Mészáros, A., & Bitter, I. (2009). Prevalence and correlates of adult attention-deficit hyperactivity disorder: Meta-analysis. *The British Journal of Psychiatry: The Journal of Mental Science*, *194*(3), 204–211. https://doi.org/10.1192/bjp.bp.107.048827

Sinha, A., Lewis, O., Kumar, R., Yeruva, S. L. H., & Curry, B. H. (2016). Adult ADHD Medications and Their

Cardiovascular Implications. *Case Reports in Cardiology,*
2016, 2343691. https://doi.org/10.1155/2016/2343691

Smith, M. E., & Farah, M. J. (2011). Are Prescription Stimulants
"Smart Pills"? *Psychological Bulletin, 137*(5), 717–741.
https://doi.org/10.1037/a0023825

Song, M., Dieckmann, N. F., & Nigg, J. T. (2019). Addressing
Discrepancies Between ADHD Prevalence and Case
Identification Estimates Among U.S. Children Utilizing
NSCH 2007-2012. *Journal of Attention Disorders, 23*(14),
1691–1702.
https://doi.org/10.1177/1087054718799930

Sprague, R. L., & Sleator, E. K. (1977). Methylphenidate in
Hyperkinetic Children: Differences in Dose Effects on
Learning and Social Behavior. *Science, 198*(4323), 1274–
1276. https://doi.org/10.1126/science.337493

Staerk, L., Wang, B., Preis, S. R., Larson, M. G., Lubitz, S. A.,
Ellinor, P. T., McManus, D. D., Ko, D., Weng, L.-C.,
Lunetta, K. L., Frost, L., Benjamin, E. J., & Trinquart, L.
(2018). Lifetime risk of atrial fibrillation according to
optimal, borderline, or elevated levels of risk factors:
Cohort study based on longitudinal data from the
Framingham Heart Study. *BMJ, 361*, k1453.
https://doi.org/10.1136/bmj.k1453

Strauss, A. A., & Lehtinen, L. E. (1947). *Psychopathology and
education of the brain-injured child* (p. 206). Grune &
Stratton.

Tait, G. (2009). The Logic of ADHD: A Brief Review of Fallacious
Reasoning. *Studies in Philosophy and Education, 28*(3),
239–254. https://doi.org/10.1007/s11217-008-9114-2

Talsma, D., Senkowski, D., Soto-Faraco, S., & Woldorff, M. G.
(2010). The multifaceted interplay between attention
and multisensory integration. *Trends in Cognitive
Sciences, 14*(9), 400–410.
https://doi.org/10.1016/j.tics.2010.06.008

Teo, S. K., Stirling, D. I., Hoberman, A. M., Christian, M. S.,
Thomas, S. D., & Khetani, V. D. (2003). D-
methylphenidate and D,L-methylphenidate are not

developmental toxicants in rats and rabbits. *Birth Defects Research. Part B, Developmental and Reproductive Toxicology, 68*(2), 162–171. https://doi.org/10.1002/bdrb.10018

Teter, C. J., McCabe, S. E., LaGrange, K., Cranford, J. A., & Boyd, C. J. (2006). Illicit use of specific prescription stimulants among college students: Prevalence, motives, and routes of administration. *Pharmacotherapy, 26*(10), 1501–1510. https://doi.org/10.1592/phco.26.10.1501

Tipper, C. M., Cairo, T. A., Woodward, T. S., Phillips, A. G., Liddle, P. F., & Ngan, E. T. C. (2005). Processing efficiency of a verbal working memory system is modulated by amphetamine: An fMRI investigation. *Psychopharmacology, 180*(4), 634–643. https://doi.org/10.1007/s00213-005-0025-4

Torres-Acosta, N., O'Keefe, J. H., O'Keefe, C. L., & Lavie, C. J. (2020). Cardiovascular Effects of ADHD Therapies: JACC Review Topic of the Week. *Journal of the American College of Cardiology, 76*(7), 858–866. https://doi.org/10.1016/j.jacc.2020.05.081

Triolo, S. J. (2001). ADHD, Evolution, and Today's Research Focus: A Response to Barkley. *The ADHD Report, 9*(4), 5–8. https://doi.org/10.1521/adhd.9.4.5.19064

Vaa, T. (2014). ADHD and relative risk of accidents in road traffic: A meta-analysis. *Accident Analysis & Prevention, 62*, 415–425. https://doi.org/10.1016/j.aap.2013.10.003

Varambally, S., Venkatasubramanian, G., & Gangadhar, B. N. (2012). Neurological soft signs in schizophrenia—The past, the present and the future. *Indian Journal of Psychiatry, 54*(1), 73–80. https://doi.org/10.4103/0019-5545.94653

Volkow, N. D., Han, B., Compton, W. M., & McCance-Katz, E. F. (2019). Self-reported Medical and Nonmedical Cannabis Use Among Pregnant Women in the United States. *JAMA, 322*(2), 167–169. https://doi.org/10.1001/jama.2019.7982

Waddington, P. (1996). *Dying for information?: An investigation into the effects of information overload in the UK and worldwide*. Reuters.

Wang, L.-J., Lee, S.-Y., Yuan, S.-S., Yang, C.-J., Yang, K.-C., Huang, T.-S., Chou, W.-J., Chou, M.-C., Lee, M.-J., Lee, T.-L., & Shyu, Y.-C. (2016). Prevalence rates of youths diagnosed with and medicated for ADHD in a nationwide survey in Taiwan from 2000 to 2011. *Epidemiology and Psychiatric Sciences*, *26*(6), 624–634. https://doi.org/10.1017/S2045796016000500

Warshak, C. R., Regan, J., Moore, B., Magner, K., Kritzer, S., & Van Hook, J. (2015). Association between marijuana use and adverse obstetrical and neonatal outcomes. *Journal of Perinatology*, *35*(12), Article 12. https://doi.org/10.1038/jp.2015.120

Webb, J. R., Valasek, M. A., & North, C. S. (2013). *Prevalence of stimulant use in a sample of US medical students. 25*(1), 27–32.

Wender, P. (1971). *Minimal Brain Dysfunction in Children*. Wiley-Interscience, A Division of John Wiley & Sons,.

Westover, A. N., & Halm, E. A. (2012). Do prescription stimulants increase the risk of adverse cardiovascular events?: A systematic review. *BMC Cardiovascular Disorders*, *12*(1), 41. https://doi.org/10.1186/1471-2261-12-41

Whalley, L. J., Dick, F. D., & McNeill, G. (2006). A life-course approach to the aetiology of late-onset dementias. *The Lancet Neurology*, *5*(1), 87–96.

Wheater, E. N. W., Shenkin, S. D., Maniega, S. M., Hernández, M. V., Wardlaw, J. M., Deary, I. J., Bastin, M. E., Boardman, J. P., & Cox, S. R. (2020). *Birth weight is associated with brain tissue volumes seven decades later, but not with age-associated changes to brain structure* (p. 2020.08.27.270033). bioRxiv. https://doi.org/10.1101/2020.08.27.270033

White, J. D. (1999). Review Personality, temperament and ADHD: A review of the literature. *Personality and*

Individual Differences, 27(4), 589–598.
https://doi.org/10.1016/S0191-8869(98)00273-6

Wilens, T. E., Adler, L. A., Adams, J., Sgambati, S., Rotrosen, J.,
Sawtelle, R., Utzinger, L., & Fusillo, S. (2008). Misuse
and diversion of stimulants prescribed for ADHD: A
systematic review of the literature. *Journal of the
American Academy of Child and Adolescent Psychiatry,
47*(1), 21–31.
https://doi.org/10.1097/chi.0b013e31815a56f1

Wilens, T. E., Hammerness, P. G., Biederman, J., Kwon, A.,
Spencer, T. J., Clark, S., Scott, M., Podolski, A., Ditterline,
J. W., Morris, M. C., & Moore, H. (2005). Blood pressure
changes associated with medication treatment of adults
with attention-deficit/hyperactivity disorder. *The
Journal of Clinical Psychiatry, 66*(2), 253–259.
https://doi.org/10.4088/jcp.v66n0215

Willcutt, E. G. (2012). The prevalence of DSM-IV attention-
deficit/hyperactivity disorder: A meta-analytic review.
*Neurotherapeutics: The Journal of the American Society
for Experimental NeuroTherapeutics, 9*(3), 490–499.
https://doi.org/10.1007/s13311-012-0135-8

Wood, S., Sage, J. R., Shuman, T., & Anagnostaras, S. G. (2014a).
Psychostimulants and cognition: A continuum of
behavioral and cognitive activation. *Pharmacological
Reviews, 66*(1), 193–221.
https://doi.org/10.1124/pr.112.007054

Wood, S., Sage, J. R., Shuman, T., & Anagnostaras, S. G. (2014b).
Psychostimulants and Cognition: A Continuum of
Behavioral and Cognitive Activation. *Pharmacological
Reviews, 66*(1), 193–221.
https://doi.org/10.1124/pr.112.007054

Wouldes, T., LaGasse, L., Sheridan, J., & Lester, B. (2004).
*Maternal methamphetamine use during pregnancy and
child outcome: What do we know? 117*(1206), 11.

Yakovlev, P. (1967). Yakovlev, Paul I. "The myelogenetic cycles
of regional maturation of the brain." Regional

development of the brain in early life (1967). In *Regional development of the brain in early life.*

Yakovlev, P. I. (1962). Morphological criteria of growth and maturation of the nervous system in man. *Research Publications - Association for Research in Nervous and Mental Disease, 39,* 3–46.

Yerys, B. E., Gordon, E. M., Abrams, D. N., Satterthwaite, T. D., Weinblatt, R., Jankowski, K. F., Strang, J., Kenworthy, L., Gaillard, W. D., & Vaidya, C. J. (2015). Default mode network segregation and social deficits in autism spectrum disorder: Evidence from non-medicated children. *NeuroImage. Clinical, 9,* 223–232. https://doi.org/10.1016/j.nicl.2015.07.018

Zullig, K. J., Divin, A. L., Weiler, R. M., Haddox, J. D., & Pealer, L. N. (2015). Adolescent Nonmedical Use of Prescription Pain Relievers, Stimulants, and Depressants, and Suicide Risk. *Substance Use & Misuse, 50*(13), 1678–1689. https://doi.org/10.3109/10826084.2015.1027931